THE FAT SMASH DIET

ALSO BY IAN K. SMITH, M.D.

The Take-Control Diet

Dr. Ian Smith's Guide to Medical Websites

The Blackbird Papers: A Novel

THE FAT SMASH DIET

• The Last Diet You'll Ever Need •

Ian K. Smith, M.D.

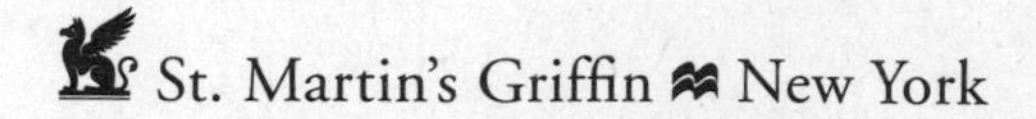
St. Martin's Griffin New York

AUTHOR'S NOTE: This book proposes a program of dietary and exercise recommendations for the reader to follow and is offered as an informational guide. However, you should consult a qualified medical professional before starting this or any other weight reduction or exercise program. As with any diet or exercise program, if at any time you experience any discomfort or have questions or concerns after embarking on the program, stop immediately and consult your physicians.

Also, reference in this book to products, service providers, and potential sources of additional information does not mean that the author or the publisher endorses such products or services or the information or recommendations in such sources. Neither the author nor the publishers are responsible for any product or service or the content or policies of any Web site or other source over which they do not have control.

www.stmartins.com
www.fatsmashdiet.com

Book design by Sita Silva of FINN Creations

Library of Congress Catalogue-in-Publication Data Available Upon Request

ISBN 0-312-36313-3
EAN 978-0-312-36316-0

Originally published in slightly different form by Health Media Strategies, LLC

10 9

To Lynn Cherry, my beautiful aunt

May you lead a longer, healthier, and happier life now that you're one hundred pounds lighter.

In the words of the great singer Barry White:

"I love you just the way you are."

THE FAT SMASH DIET

AUTHOR'S NOTE

Many of you have either seen or heard of my diet program on the popular VH1 show *Celebrity Fit Club.* Over the past year I have received thousands of e-mails from viewers asking me to share with them the diet that I have put many Hollywood celebrities on with tremendous success. I want to get something clear right from the beginning. This is not a "celebrity" diet. This is a diet for EVERYONE. It is not based on gimmicks or false promises or fake science like a lot of other programs you'll find on the market. This is a nutritionally sound, scientifically based program that if followed correctly will deliver results even to those who have not succeeded on other diets.

With many years of experience working with tens of thousands of dieters, I have learned as much from the people who are trying to lose weight as they have learned from me. One of my biggest lessons—most dieters want a simple, easy-to-follow, realistic plan that does not require a tremendous expenditure of money or time. Dieters want to be able to eat reasonably, which means enjoying an ice cream cone or a couple of chocolate chip cookies or a slice of pizza every so often. It's ridiculous to think that people are going to go through the rest of their life without having a slice of cake for dessert or a drink of alcohol when socializing with family and friends. What I've learned is that if a meal plan includes a good percentage of "likeable" foods, then people are much more willing to stick to that program than a program that eliminates all of the "fun" foods and makes unrealistic dietary demands.

I followed the advice and lessons I've gotten from thousands of dieters living all over the world. These pages are full of *only* relevant information, as I have—excuse the pun—trimmed the fat to give you just the essentials that you will need to be successful. I created The **FAT SMASH DIET** as an answer to all of the diet questions I've received over the years and the pleas from people who are simply fed up with being overweight. The **FAT SMASH DIET** is easy to follow, inexpensive, forgiving, and healthy. You will get as much out of it as you put into it. It has worked for not only Hollywood celebrities, but my friends and family members who couldn't believe they lost so much weight while still eating many of the foods they have always enjoyed.

You too can finally shed the weight and start feeling good about yourself both on the outside and inside. Remember, if you cheat, you're only cheating yourself. But if you follow the program and remain dedicated, you will be transformed into a new you, ready to take advantage of all the great things that life has to offer.

Enjoy!

—Dr. Ian Smith
New York City
January 2006

CHAPTER 1
The FAT SMASH DIET Philosophy

Diets don't fail people; people fail diets. The **FAT SMASH DIET** is a program that will never fail you if you open your mind to the great possibilities, believe in yourself, and give a full commitment. The **FAT SMASH DIET** is designed to be a forgiving program that is as much about helping people make the necessary lifestyle changes to lead a healthier, happier, and longer life as it is about getting rid of extra weight that only increases your odds of developing devastating medical complications such as high blood pressure, diabetes, and heart disease. I'm a realist. Most people have a difficult time following diets to the letter, slipping every once in a while when they can't resist the urges or when they've reached a plateau and feel like the weight is no longer coming off. The **FAT SMASH DIET** understands this and allows you to dial back into the program if necessary, by returning to Phase I, getting back on course, then resuming the program where you left off.

The **FAT SMASH DIET** is a 90-day program with four phases that will ultimately re-wire your body and its relationship to food and physical activity for the rest of your life. This is not about short-term fixes that will eventually fade and put you back where you started. Instead, this is about life change for the long term! At the end of the 90 days, you will have made small but important adjustments not only in your food consumption, but in your understanding and attitude towards food and the way you view the role of physical activity in maintaining a healthy life. Each phase builds upon the previous phase like the levels of a pyramid that support the ones above it. The foundation and its integrity are what allow the peak to stand, so you must be careful in constructing the building blocks. A strong foundation will allow you to reach the top of your goals.

I have been shocked reading many diet books that say exercising is unnecessary or it's optional based on a dieter's preferences. One of the major reasons why so many people are overweight and obese and dying from preventable medical conditions such as heart disease is because we have become too sedentary! There are numerous studies from the best researchers in the world that show how important being physically active is not just for losing weight, but becoming healthier and protecting things like our blood vessels, lungs, and heart.

Studies also show that those who incorporate a regular exercise program in their schedule will not only lose more weight faster, but will keep it off for longer periods of time. The problem that most people have is that they associate exercising with going to the gym and killing themselves for two hours, then dragging themselves home exhausted. That's *not* the exercise I'm talking about. Let's be realistic. It's not like you're training to become an Olympic gold medalist, right? What you need is a regular program of physical activity that will keep your heart rate up and your lungs working. This will also help to tone your muscles and keep your joints active to help prevent certain illnesses like the dreaded arthritis. For each phase I give you very simple exercise suggestions to help you on your journey of becoming healthier and slimmer. Choose those exercises that you like and try to find a partner who is willing to do them with you. Studies have also shown that those who are most successful at losing weight have some type of support system in place—and a weight-loss partner makes exercise more fun!

The **FAT SMASH DIET** is about smashing the bad habits and demons of the past and constructing a new and improved you now ready to take on fresh challenges and passions while fully enjoying the gift of life. Let's be perfectly clear. Diets are not magic. They are only blueprints. If you carefully follow the blueprint, then what you build can be magnificent. The **FAT SMASH DIET** is a blueprint that will help people trying to lose just 10 pounds as well as people trying to lose 200 pounds. I'm extremely proud of this program because it teaches the correct principles of healthy eating while at the same time allowing you to have a slice of cake or a couple of scoops of ice cream every now and again. Almost everything in life is about finding a balance and doing things in moderation. These are the underlying principles of The **FAT SMASH DIET**. You now are a SMASHER, so go SMASH IT!

Chapter 2

Phase I: DETOX (*9 days*)

This phase is ground zero, the beginning of the journey. The name "detox" pretty much says it all. For the next 9 days, you will eat mostly fruits and veggies and clean your body and mind of impurities naturally without fasting or putting any toxins into your system. This is about purifying your body and blood and feeding them the nutrients, vitamins, and minerals that they so badly need. It's also about opening your mind and freeing it from the imprisonment of an unhealthy lifestyle that might be holding you back from reaching your peak. This is the first step towards a new you, so it's critical that you follow the principles of this phase and don't stray from the course.

Start by weighing yourself in the nude or a swimming suit the morning you start this phase, then don't weigh yourself again until the morning of day 10. Have someone photograph you in a bathing suit. Take three shots with your hands hanging freely by your sides—a frontal shot, one taken from the side, and the third from behind. Don't suck in your stomach or assume any unnatural poses. Just stand there and be real.

You need to record your healthy weight range, something that's indicated by your Body Mass Index (BMI). (You can find out how to do this in the appendix.) This is the measurement doctors now use to determine what you should weigh for your particular height.

Surround yourself with positive energy and people who are supportive and respectful of your new journey. Reduce stressful occurrences in your life: Stress only distracts you from your important missions and induces poor decisions. Try not to think about food and weight constantly! There's a lot more to life than food and worrying about the numbers on an inanimate scale. Take up a hobby and keep busy with the fun things in life. This will help the time fly and keep you energized. If your mind isn't in the right place, then you won't be able to lose weight. Dieting is 50% mental. Don't forget that!

And remember, cheating is a decision. If cheating is the choice you make, you are only cheating yourself. Now let's start SMASHING!

NUMBER OF MEALS PER DAY: (*4-5*)

These meals are designed in moderately sized portions. Don't stuff your plate as if you won't ever get to eat again. Now that you're eating more meals, you'll have less down time between meals, and you'll experience fewer hunger pangs. Because you'll be eating every 3-4 hours, you don't need to eat so much at each meal. It's important that you understand this. Even if you're not hungry, it's **critical** that you don't skip meals. Just eat a lighter meal. Your body needs to get into a comfortable and reliable routine where it expects to be properly nourished at consistent time intervals.

QUANTITY OF FRUITS AND VEGGIES:

Eat the amount that fills you up. There is no limit and there's no counting calories. But even with this freedom, don't overeat! It's a bad habit and unnecessary. You'll be eating again soon enough. Keep in mind portion control at all times!

MYTH:

If I skip meals or only eat once a day, I will lose weight because I'm eating fewer calories.

TRUTH:

The act of eating actually increases your metabolism, which helps you burn off the calories and lose weight. When you don't eat, your body goes into "starvation mode," which means your metabolism slows down tremendously and the calories that you do ingest are automatically stored as fat. The body does this because fat is a great reserve of potential energy and can supply us in the future when this energy is needed. When you skip meals and "starve" yourself, the body doesn't know when it might see more food energy again, so it conserves and holds on to whatever it does see, storing it in the form of fat.

FOOD PREPARATION:

Foods are ONLY to be eaten raw, grilled, or steamed. You're allowed 3 tablespoons of low-fat dressing on your salads. If you're grilling the veggies, use a minimal amount of virgin olive oil (one to two teaspoons).

SAMPLE SCHEDULE:

Note: This is just a sample. You have to work out a schedule that fits your lifestyle, but keep in mind the spacing of the meals and the need to at least have 4 meals per day. For late-night snacks, try sliced fruit or raw/ steamed veggies like celery, carrots, cucumbers, broccoli, or asparagus.

8 am ....Meal #1

11 am ....Meal #2 *(heavy snack)*

2 pm ....Meal #3

5 pm ....Meal #4 *(light snack)*

7 pm ....Meal #5

9 pm ....Light Snack

DR. IAN'S TIP #1: Try frozen seedless grapes. Put the grapes in the freezer, then grab them as you like. They're delicious and low in calories!

DR. IAN'S TIP #2: Never eat within an hour and a half of going to bed. Try going for at least a 20 or 25-minute walk after dinner or participate in some other type of physical activity. This will help rev up your metabolism and burn off those calories before going to bed. It also releases endorphins, special chemicals in the body that make you feel good!

DR. IAN'S TIP #3: Eat foods high in fiber. Studies have shown that fiber helps to make you feel full longer, delays hunger pangs, reduces cholesterol levels, reduces constipation, reduces the risk of heart disease, and potentially helps prevent some intestinal cancers. Dietary sources of fiber include whole grains, fruits, vegetables, nuts, and seeds.

FOOD/DRINKS ALLOWED: *(Phase I)*

- All fruits in any quantity
- All vegetables in any quantity, *except*:

  NO white potatoes

  NO avocados
- Good sources of protein:

  chickpeas

  beans

  tofu

  lentils
- Brown rice—2 cups of cooked rice per day
- 2 cups of low-fat or skim or soy milk per day
- As much water as you like!
- Oatmeal—1 cup per day
- All herbs and spices
- 6 oz. low-fat yogurt (2 times per day)
- 4 egg whites per day
- 2 cups of herbal tea per day

FOOD/DRINKS NOT ALLOWED:
(Phase I)

- White rice
- Meat
- Fish
- Cheese
- Bread—all types
- Raisins
- Nuts
- Dried or preserved fruits
- Candy/popcorn/chips
- Ice cream
- Alcohol
- Juice
- Soda—regular *or* diet
- Coffee and all coffee drinks
- Sports drinks
- Milkshakes
- Whole eggs or yolks
- Fried food
- Fast food

PHYSICAL ACTIVITY

At least 30 minutes of cardiovascular activity five days a week.

SAMPLE ACTIVITIES:	AMOUNT OF CALORIES (*Burned Per Hour*)
Pilates (light)	200
Pilates (moderate)	300
Elliptical machine (moderate)	300
Tennis (singles)	350
Pilates (intense)	400
Kickboxing	400–600
Dancing (aerobic)	420
Bicycle riding (moderate)	450
Power walking (3 mph)	450
Aerobics	450
Jogging (5 mph)	500

Swimming (active) 500

Hiking 500

Rowing (moderate effort) 550

Power Walking (intense effort)......................... 600

Basketball 700

Rowing (intense effort) 700

Running (11 to 30–min. mile) 700

Jump rope (moderate—70 jumps / min) 700

Elliptical machine (intense) 700

Jump rope (intense—125 jumps / min) 850

Running (10–min. mile) 850

Stair climbing (stadiums) 900

STRUCTURE: AT LEAST 30 minutes 5 days a week. You can choose any five days you like. They don't have to be consecutive and can include all, part, or none of the weekend. It's also fine to do more days if you like. Anything over five is bonus! Keep a simple journal of the type of physical activity you engaged in, the time of day you did it, and the amount of time you spent doing it.

SAMPLE SCHEDULE:

MON.	30 minutes—power walking (300 cal.)
TUES.	OFF DAY
WED.	30 minutes—elliptical (350 cal.)
THURS.	30 minutes—aerobics (225 cal.)
FRI.	OFF DAY
SAT.	30 minutes—stair climbing (450 cal.)
SUN.	30 minutes—cycling (225 cal.)

DR IAN'S TIP #4: Try to get your workout done early in the morning. It's a great start to the day and it takes the pressure off later, when you might be tired from a full day of work or busy with other plans. Also, if you work out early in the morning, you can always do some type of physical activity at night for a bonus!

DR. IAN'S TIP #5: While it's faster and more organized to meet your physical activity component by working out in a gym, you don't have to belong to a gym to make this program work. Not everyone likes gyms and they can be costly. Try stair climbs or mini stadiums. Go up and down a flight of stairs of at least 10 steps. Up and back down is considered 1 trip. Try to do at least 10 trips within 30 minutes with 30 to 45-second rest periods between each trip. If you don't want to make noise in the house, go to the local high school track and use the bleachers. This is a GREAT workout and it doesn't cost anything.

DR. IAN'S TIP #6: CARDIO FAT BURNING

Work out with your heart rate in the fat-burning zone: 50-70% of maximum heart rate. Subtract your age from 220 to find your maximum heart rate. Then multiply that number by .50—this will give you the minimum heart rate you should maintain while performing your physical activity. Then take your maximum heart rate and multiply it by .70—this is the upper range for maximal fat burning.

EXAMPLE: (*40-year-old person*)

220 - 40 = 180 (maximum heart rate)

180 x .50 = 90 (lower limit of minimal fat-burning range)

180 x .70 = 126 (upper limit of maximal fat-burning range)

Range during exercise for maximal fat burning: 90-126 beats per minute

NOTE: THOSE WHO ARE BETTER CONDITIONED SHOULD WORK WITHIN THE RANGE OF 60-75% OF MAXIMUM HEART RATE.

Chapter 3
Phase II: FOUNDATION
(3 weeks)

CONGRATULATIONS! You have gone through the most difficult part of the program: detoxification. Now that your body has detoxed and you have reintroduced the nourishing powers of fruits and vegetables to your diet, it's time to start laying the foundation to a healthier way of eating and a healthier you.

The purpose of this phase is to reintroduce many foods you missed during detox, those very foods your body was craving to eat. At this point it's important to remember that this is about SMASHING those bad habits of the past and building good habits for the future. It's important to stick to the guidelines of the program with an understanding that you and your eating program are a work in progress. Now is not the time to undo all of the progress you've made in Phase I, so some of the basic rules still apply: (1) do not overeat at any given sitting, but maintain the schedule of 4-5 smaller meals per day; (2) continue to eat as many fruits and vegetables as possible even though you are adding other foods to your diet; (3) DON'T skip meals and stick as closely as possible to the eating schedule that you've set up in Phase I, since this is what your body is now accustomed to following; (4) you MUST continue the physical activity portion of the program as this will be the best way that you continue to burn off those calories and SMASH the fat; (5) continue to stay away from fried foods and fat-laden dressings that only add unnecessary calories and distribute bad fats in your blood.

Remember, we are building that pyramid and in order for the peak to tower beautifully in the sky, the blocks upon which it rests must remain strong and dependable. The blocks you put down in this phase are the most important since they are your FOUNDATION. Go SMASH it!

NUMBER OF MEALS PER DAY: (*4-5*)

It's EXTREMELY important that you eat at least 4 meals a day, because we are now adding more fun foods back in the diet and these fun foods pack a lot more calories than the fruits and vegetables of Phase I. Eating multiple meals will reduce the time you're waiting between meals and will help you to continue to cut down on the hunger pangs and cravings. Remember, it's all about smashing bad habits and building new ones. Setting a regular eating schedule is an important habit to develop! Maintain the smaller portions!

QUANTITY OF FRUITS AND VEGGIES:

As in the previous phase, there's no limit to the amount of fruits and veggies you can eat at each meal, with the exception of avocados and potatoes. Remember, this is a diet where you don't have to sit down with a calculator and figure out how many calories you're consuming. Let hunger be your guide. Eat the fruits and veggies until the hunger is gone, but DON'T eat so much that you get up from the table feeling stuffed. This is essential. You will be re-energizing yourself in no more than a few hours, so don't overdo it in one sitting.

FOOD/DRINKS ALLOWED: *(Phase II)*

Vegetables and grains:

- Bok choy
- Broccoli
- Collard greens
- Dark green leafy lettuce
- Kale
- Mesclun
- Romaine lettuce
- Spinach
- Watercress
- Acorn squash
- Butternut squash
- Carrots
- Pumpkin
- Sweet potatoes
- Black beans
- Black-eyed peas
- Chickpeas
- Kidney beans
- Lentils
- Corn
- Green peas

- Lima beans
- Artichokes
- Asparagus
- Bean sprouts
- Beets
- Brussel sprouts
- Cabbage
- Cauliflower
- Celery
- Cucumbers
- Eggplant
- Green beans
- Green/red peppers
- Mushrooms
- Okra
- Onions
- Parsnips
- Tomatoes
- Brown rice—2 cups of cooked rice *every other day (if desired)*
- Avocado—1/2 per day maximum

NEW **NOTE: These are total servings allowed per day; eat your servings during any meal you choose.**

MEATS *3-4 oz.* (size of a deck of playing cards)	Chicken: baked without the skin (NO FRIED!) Turkey: baked without the skin Ground beef: EXTRA lean or ground sirloin, broiled Sirloin steak, broiled Lamb, broiled
SEAFOOD	Halibut, Tuna, Salmon, Snapper, Striped Bass, etc.: 3 oz. (NO FRIED!) Shrimp: 4 large Mussels: 3 oz. Oysters: 6-12 Clams: 3
EGGS	4 egg whites *plus* 1 whole egg—scrambled, boiled, or poached
MILK & CHEESE	2½ cups of low-fat, skim, or soy milk Cheese: 1 oz. (about 1.5 slices) 6 oz. low-fat yogurt (2 times per day)

>>

CEREALS cold unsweetened *1½ cups per day* hot *½ cup per day*	Corn flakes Cheerios Oatmeal Farina/Cream of wheat Total Bran flakes Life Rice Crispies Puffed rice Puffed wheat Shredded wheat Wheaties Special K Chex
SWEETENERS	4 tsp of granulated sugar (or sugar substitute)
SPICES & HERBS as you like!	Salt (2 tsp) Pepper (as you like)

>>

FLAVORINGS	2 tbsp of fat-free dressing Extra virgin olive oil—1 tbsp 1 tbsp of fat-free mayo 2 pats of butter (two teaspoons)
DRINKS	1 10-oz. cup of coffee 3 cups of tea 5 cups of club soda 2 cans of diet soda 1 cup of freshly squeezed fruit juice (you can divide this up into ½ cup servings) Iced tea—sweetened only with 2 packets of sugar substitute Lemonade—made with real lemons and 2 packets of sugar substitute or 2 tsp of granulated sugar Flavored seltzer or tonic water unlimited Unlimited tap or bottled water!

FOOD/DRINKS NOT ALLOWED:

(Phase II)

- White rice
- White potatoes
- Bread/English muffins
- White pasta or whole wheat pasta
- White flour
- Pastries/donuts/Danish
- Cake
- Cookies
- Brownies
- Candy
- Ice cream
- Potato chips/corn chips/ Tortilla chips/popcorn
- Chocolate
- Bacon
- Sausage
- Alcohol
- Fried food
- Fast food

>>

>>

- Regular soda
- Sweetened juices from a bottle or can
- Milkshakes
- Frappuccinos
- Café latte or cappuccino

TIPS:

- Don't eat the same fish or meat twice in the same day
- Try to separate the meats by at least a meal
- Try to leave some of the food on your plate when you get up from the table
- Try to do some physical activity after eating dinner (at least 20 minutes)
- Only snack on fruits and veggies after dinner
- Remember portion size: less is more!

PHYSICAL ACTIVITY:

Same program as Phase I, except it's time to KICK IT UP because you're now eating a lot more calories, so you must increase everything by 10-15 %.

For example: If you had walked for 30 minutes a day, now walk for 35.

If you walked a mile a day, now walk 1.1-1.2 miles.

Remember, do the cardio exercises in your heart range, which was explained in Phase I (page 27).

The more you do the better!

No lifting free weights! (This will come in Phase III or IV)

SAMPLE SCHEDULE:

MON.	35 minutes—elliptical (408 cal.)
TUES.	35 minutes—swimming (291 cal.)
WED.	OFF DAY
THURS.	35 minutes—power walking (intense) (350 cal.)
FRI.	OFF DAY
SAT.	35 minutes—aerobics (263 cal.)
SUN.	35 minutes—jumping rope (408 cal.)

Chapter 4
Phase III: CONSTRUCTION
(*4 weeks*)

Over the last four weeks, you have laid down a solid foundation for a healthier lifestyle that we will now continue to build on. Phase III will add more variety to your diet, constructing an eating plan that will allow you to enjoy many of the foods you've enjoyed in the past. The difference, however, is that with your greater understanding of portion control and the importance of more fruits and vegetables in your diet, you can now enjoy some of those sweets you've missed in the past, but instead of eating five cookies, you'll be content with two. The first two phases instilled some important concepts that will guide your eating behaviors forever. Don't turn your back on all that you have learned and take up the old bad habits. Doing this will reverse the progress you've worked so hard to make.

Remember that you are now eating AT LEAST four times a day, which means you don't have to fill your plate to the rim, go back for seconds, or eat super-sized meals. Your body is now accustomed to consistency: the regular schedule of your eating times and the volume of food that you're consuming at one sitting. Do the best that you can not to disrupt this schedule, but if for some reason you can't maintain it, go back to it as soon as possible. A short interruption will not throw you too far off course. No dieter is perfect and at some point it is very likely that you might slip. This is not uncommon. It happens to almost everyone. If you slip, don't get anxious. The **FAT SMASH DIET** is designed to forgive, not punish. Simply go back on Phase I until you've lost any weight you have gained back. Once you've lost that weight, go an extra day on Phase I, then directly back to Phase III.

NUMBER OF MEALS PER DAY: (*4-5*)

QUANTITY OF FRUITS AND VEGGIES:

Let hunger be your guide. Eat enough that you're satisfied, not so much that you're stuffed. Remember these foods are most nutritious when they're eaten raw, steamed, grilled, or baked. Frying is not permitted since this adds extra calories and destroys the nutrients contained in the food.

DR. IAN'S TIP **:** Try one day of Phase I during each week of Phase III. This will cut the calories down for a few days and shake your body from its comfortable routine, which can kick-start more weight loss.

FOOD/DRINKS ALLOWED: *(Phase III)*

Vegetables and grains:

- Bok choy
- Broccoli
- Collard greens
- Dark green leafy lettuce
- Kale
- Mesclun
- Romaine lettuce
- Spinach
- Watercress
- Acorn squash
- Butternut squash
- Carrots
- Pumpkin
- Sweet potatoes
- Black beans
- Black-eyed peas
- Chickpeas
- Kidney beans
- Lentils
- Corn

- Green peas
- Lima beans
- Artichokes
- Asparagus
- Bean sprouts
- Beets
- Brussel sprouts
- Cabbage
- Cauliflower
- Celery
- Cucumbers
- Eggplant
- Green beans
- Green/red peppers
- Mushrooms
- Okra
- Onions
- Parsnips
- Tomatoes
- Brown rice—2 cups of
  cooked rice
  every other day (if desired)
- Avocado—1/2 per day maximum

CEREALS cold unsweetened *1½ cups per day* hot *½ cup per day*	Corn flakes Cheerios Oatmeal Farina/Cream of wheat Total Bran flakes Life Rice Crispies Puffed rice Puffed wheat Shredded wheat Wheaties Special K Chex
SWEETENERS	4 tsp of granulated sugar (or sugar substitute)
SPICES **&** **HERBS** as you like!	Salt (2 tsp) Pepper (as you like)

FLAVORINGS	2 tbsp of fat-free dressing Extra virgin olive oil—1 tbsp 1 tbsp of fat-free mayo 2 pats of butter
DRINKS	1 10-oz. cup of regular coffee 3 cups of tea 5 cups of club soda 2 cans of diet soda Iced tea—sweetened only with 2 packets of sugar substitute Lemonade—made with real lemons and 2 packets of sugar substitute or 2 tsp of granulated sugar Flavored seltzer or tonic water unlimited Unlimited tap or bottled water!

NEW

- 2 cups of freshly squeezed fruit juice (you can divide this up throughout the day as you like)

NEW **NOTE: These are total servings allowed per day; eat your servings during any meal you choose; the meat serving is now larger.**

MEATS *5 oz.* size of a deck and a half of playing cards	Chicken: baked without the skin (NO FRIED!) Turkey: baked without the skin Ground beef: EXTRA lean or ground sirloin Sirloin steak, broiled Lamb, broiled Turkey Sausage—1 link
SEAFOOD	Halibut, Tuna, Salmon, Snapper, Striped Bass, etc.: 3 oz. (NO FRIED!) Shrimp: 4 large Mussels: 3 oz. Oysters: 6-12 Clams: 3
EGGS	4 egg whites *plus* 2 whole eggs—scrambled, boiled, or poached
MILK & CHEESE	3 cups of low-fat, skim, or soy milk Cheese: 1.3 oz. (about 2 slices)

PASTA & BREAD	Whole wheat pasta: 1 cup per day Whole wheat/whole grain bread: 4 thin slices
DESSERTS the serving size for the cookies is approximately the size of a silver dollar (*e.g., an Oreo*)	Note: *One dessert per day at any meal you choose.* 3 chocolate chip cookes 4 gingersnaps 2 oatmeal raisin cookes 2 peanut butter cookes 2 whole graham crackers 1 scoop of low-fat ice cream

FOOD/DRINKS NOT ALLOWED:

(Phase III)

- White rice
- White potatoes
- White bread/English muffins
- White pasta
- White flour
- Pastries/donuts/Danish
- Cake
- Brownies
- Candy
- Potato chips/corn chips/ tortilla chips/popcorn
- Bacon
- Sausage
- Alcohol
- Regular sodas
- Milkshakes
- Frappuccinos or cappuccinos
- Café latte

PHYSICAL ACTIVITY:

Same program as Phase II, except it's time to kick it up again; you're now eating a lot more calories, so you must increase everything by 25%.

For example: if you were walking for 35 minutes a day, now walk for 45.

If you walked 1.1 miles a day, now walk 1.4 miles a day

Remember, do the cardio exercises in your heart range, which was explained in Phase I. (page 27)

Light free weights are optional, but it's better to do them in the next phase.

DR. IAN'S TIP **:** Try to burn off some extra calories by doing a "two-a-day." This is what many well-conditioned athletes do. Work out twice in one day: a morning exercise routine and another in the evening. This will really rev up your metabolism.

SAMPLE SCHEDULE:

MON.	OFF DAY
TUES.	45 minutes—aerobics (338 cal.)
WED.	45 minutes—elliptical (525 cal.)
THURS.	OFF DAY
FRI.	45 minutes—basketball, full court (525 cal.)
SAT.	45 minutes—swimming (375 cal.)
SUN.	45 minutes—stair climbing (675 cal.)

Chapter 5
Phase IV: THE TEMPLE
(*for life*)

The fact that you've made it to this phase means that you have achieved tremendous success. This is no small feat. Be proud of yourself! You have **detoxed** your body, laid a solid **foundation** for a healthier way of living, and **constructed** a routine of good habits that will guide you throughout your life. All of this is like building a sacred temple, something to admire, respect, and honor. But like any beautiful structure, there's also maintenance involved to keep it clean and shiny. Every once in a while there will be the need for minor repairs, and that's expected. The key, however, is to avoid the need for major fixes. This is where you are on The **FAT SMASH DIET**. Now that you've built the temple of good eating behaviors and a physical activity program, you can admire and appreciate it, but also be prepared for minor tweaks as you go along. Remember that life is constantly evolving.

This phase is fluid in nature, since you never know

where the repairs need to be done or when. Maybe you've started eating too many sweets or increased the portions beyond the appropriate sizes. Some people will start slacking off on the physical activity regimen and will notice the weight slowly starting to creep back on. Don't get upset or frustrated. These are not major problems and they can be addressed very easily. That's the beauty of The **FAT SMASH DIET**. The important part is to identify the exact location of the leak in the roof and quickly use the necessary material to fix it. If you notice that you've gained back 10-15% of the weight that you had lost earlier, then simply leave the temple (Phase IV), go back to detox (Phase I) until you've lost that weight again, then return directly to Phase IV, being mindful of your portions and keeping up your physical activity.

In this last phase, there are some food and beverage additions for you that will complete your eating program. Since they've been absent from your diet for the last eight weeks, you can better appreciate them, but it's important to follow the guidelines and not overindulge. Remember, at this stage of the diet, you have SMASHED the bad habits and developed good, healthy habits through hard work and determination. This healthier way of living can sustain you as a lean, fit, healthy person forever.

DR. IAN'S TIP : Buy an inexpensive pedometer to keep track of how many steps you take per day. Try 6,000 steps for good health and 10,000 steps for weight loss.

NEW **NOTE: The foods from all of the previous phases are allowed in this phase. Just add from the chart below. Enjoy, but remember *PORTION CONTROL!***

BREAKFAST	Bacon—4 strips per week Sausage—2 links per week 6 4-inch pancakes per week (whole wheat is better) 1 6-inch waffle per week
LUNCH & DINNER	2 slices of cheese pizza with any toppings—twice a week White rice—2 servings a week (but brown is still better) 1 white baked potato a week (but sweet potato is still better) 2 small servings of french fries per week 1 serving of ricotta cheese 3 times per week Provolone, Swiss, or Muenster cheese, 2 slices per day 2 medium-sized crab cakes per week 1 medium-sized lobster per week (use butter sparingly!) 4 medium slices of ham per week (avoid the fat)

➤➤

DRINKS	
	2 8-oz. cups of soda per week (diet soda is much better)
	2-3 beers per week (preferably not at one sitting)
	3 glasses of wine per week (preferably not at one sitting)
	3 8-oz. café lattes or cappuccinos per week (try using fat-free milk)
	1 12-oz. milkshake per week

PHYSICAL ACTIVITY:

By this point you should be in a comfortable excercise routine. Exercise 5 times a week for 1 intense hour each time. It's very important to change your workout routine, since your body can quickly become accustomed to your exercise schedule and stop burning the calories.

Also, start lifting light free weights under supervision. This will help build up your lean muscle mass. You should lift weights at least twice a week, working on your different body parts. You can do this right at home with dumbbells. But you should make sure you have been trained on the proper lifting techniques before attempting them.

Continuing your physical activity plan is ESSENTIAL for you to develop the complete package. It will only boost the results you obtain on the diet!

Chapter 6
BUSTING THROUGH THE PLATEAU

Almost everyone over the course of a diet hits a plateau, a point where they can't seem to lose weight any more despite their previous success. This is what I call the critical point. It's critical, because unfortunately, most people get frustrated and disappointed and quit. DON'T QUIT! Plateaus are very natural and happen for a good reason. The body is an extremely clever machine and while we think that we can fool it, we can only do so for short periods of time at most. The body becomes accustomed to your new way of eating and your exercise regimen and decides that it is not going to keep burning calories by shedding fat. Believe it or not, that's an important protective feature of how our bodies operate. Imagine if you were stuck on a cold mountain with no way of getting food or water for a prolonged period of time. The body works to conserve your fat—the source of energy—as long as possible so that you can last without food and water until a rescue team arrives. Well, it's that feature that kicks in when you've been doing so well losing weight.

But there is a way to bust through this "standstill" point and it requires patience and determination. First, each time you exercise, increase it by 20% and do this for 9 days. For example, if you normally walk for 60 minutes during your exercise time, walk for 72 minutes instead. If you normally walk 2 miles at a time, walk 2.4 miles. At the same time, decrease the amount of calories you consume by eating smaller portions. This way, you're attacking the problem from both ends.

Another method is to change your diet altogether. Sometimes you have to "shock" the system to get it going. So go back to an earlier phase like I or II or a combination of them and stay there for 7 days. You can play with the combination as you like, but the idea is to do something different from what you've been doing. You should also change your exercise program. Try to do a different exercise. If you spend most of your time walking, then try doing stairs or playing a sport. Don't decrease your time, just switch up the activity.

The bottom line is that in order to bust through the plateau, you must shake your body out of its comfort zone. Do this for 7-9 days and you will get through it. There's no universal solution that works for everyone, but I have found these strategies to be very effective for most dieters I've helped over the years.

SAMPLE SCHEDULE:

MON.	60 minutes—elliptical (700 cal.)
TUES.	60 minutes—swimming (500 cal.)
WED.	OFF DAY
THURS.	60 minutes—power walking (intense) (600 cal.)
FRI.	OFF DAY
SAT.	60 minutes—aerobics (450 cal.)
SUN.	60 minutes—jumping rope, 70 jumps /min (700 cal.)

Chapter 7
TASTY RECIPES

* *Most recipes provided by Big City Chefs:* 1-866-321-CHEF **www.bigcitychefs.com**

NOTE: Look carefully at the serving sizes for the different recipes. In many cases it's 4 or more for that particular recipe, which means you are not to eat all of it. You are still ONLY to have 1 serving size per meal at most! Remember, this is about portion control. You are eating more meals per day, which means each meal MUST be smaller or you'll be packing on too many calories! Stow away the extra portions in individual containers for later in the week or stash them in the freezer for the next phase of the program.

For those readers who may lack the time or ability to prepare the recipes in this book, or for those who may enjoy an additional selection of recipes consistent with Dr. Ian's nutritional guidelines, contact Big City Chefs at 1-866-321-CHEF or at www.bigcitychefs.com. Big City Chefs staffs professionally trained personal chefs in major metropolitan regions nationwide, providing personalized menu planning and in-home preparation of one to two weeks of meals per visit.

PHASE I | Sample Recipes

GOOD BREAKFAST HABITS

BAD BREAKFAST HABITS

Breakfast | (*Phase I*)

Recipes on the go!

- ½ cup oatmeal
  1 cup of raspberries
  1 cup low-fat milk

- ½ cantaloupe
  6-oz. cup low-fat yogurt
  1 cup of fresh orange juice

- 4 egg whites
  ½ red grapefruit
  1 cup of low-fat milk

Green Bean Salad

Serves : 4-6

1 lb fresh green beans, trimmed
10 cherry tomatoes, halved
1 yellow bell pepper, seeded and julienned
½ cup chopped green bell pepper
¼ cup chopped fresh parsley

For dressing :
1 tsp Dijon mustard
¼ cup olive oil
¼ cup fresh lemon juice
¼ tsp freshly ground pepper
⅛ tsp salt

DIRECTIONS

Wash green beans thoroughly. Drop the green beans into a saucepan of boiling water. Cook until slightly crisp, about four minutes.

Drain off water and let beans cool. Add tomatoes, peppers, and parsley.

To make the dressing: Combine mustard, oil, and lemon juice in a small bowl. Stir well.

Then add pepper and salt and stir again.

Lightly pour the dressing over the salad, then toss. Transfer the salad to a serving bowl, cover, and refrigerate for at least an hour until well chilled.

Vigorous Vegetable Soup

Serves : 4

1 medium zucchini, chopped
1 cup chopped mushrooms
1 medium onion, diced
7 large carrots, diced
4 celery stalks, diced
1 sprig rosemary
1 tsp dried thyme
1 bay leaf
¼ tsp crushed red pepper flakes
1 10-oz. package frozen
green peas, thawed
3 14.5-ounce cans low-fat,
low-sodium beef broth
(or vegetable broth)
3 cups water

DIRECTIONS

Place all the ingredients except the peas in a large pot with the water, broth, and spices.

Bring to a boil, then let simmer for 45 minutes or until carrots are tender. Add peas for last 5 minutes of cooking time.

Remove the bay leaf and rosemary sprig before serving.

Carrot Soup

Serves : 4

1 tsp butter
10 carrots, chopped
1 small onion, chopped
5 cups (40 oz) of vegetable broth or beef broth
3 tbsp curry powder
¼ cup brown rice (optional)
1 tbsp minced ginger
2 cloves garlic, minced
Sprig of parsley
Bay leaves
Salt and pepper

DIRECTIONS

Melt butter in medium skillet. Add carrots and onion and sauté until soft, approximately 10-15 minutes.

Next add the remaining ingredients, bring to a boil, and simmer for 30-40 minutes.

Remove parsley and bay leaves, then pour mix into a blender in batches and puree.

Serve hot or cold.

Lentils with Grilled Mushrooms, Asparagus, and Asparagus Broth

Serves : 4

2 cups mushrooms
3 tbsp olive oil
3 cups cooked lentils
1 clove garlic, minced
1 cup steamed and chopped asparagus
2 tbsp fresh basil, cut into chiffonade (thin strips)
Salt and pepper to taste

For asparagus broth :

2 tsp olive oil
¼ cup each diced carrot, onion, and celery
2 cloves garlic, whole
2 tbsp white wine
½ cup asparagus ends, roughly chopped (*use leftover woody ends of stems that are not used above*)
3 cups vegetable broth
1 bay leaf
Basil stems *(from basil above)*
Salt and pepper to taste

DIRECTIONS

To make the asparagus broth : Heat olive oil over medium heat and sweat carrot, onion, celery, and garlic cloves for approximately 2 minutes. Add white wine and cook for 1 minute. Add asparagus ends, broth, bay leaf, and basil stems. Reduce heat and simmer for 20 minutes. Strain and set aside.

Toss mushrooms with 2 tablespoons of the olive oil and grill them on medium heat for 2 minutes per side (you may alternately oven-roast them on a baking sheet for 10 minutes at 400°F). Let mushrooms cool, then slice. Heat 1 tbsp olive oil in a sauté pan over high heat, add garlic, and briefly sweat until aromas are released. Add lentils, mushrooms, and asparagus and cook for 1 minute over high heat. Add asparagus broth and bring to a simmer. Heat through until all ingredients are hot. Remove from the heat, add the fresh basil, season to taste with salt and pepper, and serve.

NUTRITIONAL INFORMATION:

Per Serving : 417 Calories; 14g Fat (29.2% calories from fat); 20g Protein; 56g Carbohydrate; 16g Dietary Fiber; 2mg Cholesterol; 1235mg Sodium. Exchanges: 3 Grain(Starch); 1 Lean Meat; 1 Vegetable; 3 Fat.

Corn Salad

Serves : 4

3	portobello mushrooms, chopped
⅓	cup balsamic vinegar
⅓	cup olive oil
4	tsp water
	Pinch of brown or white sugar
½	pound sweet yellow corn
1	cup grape tomatoes, halved
1	medium onion, chopped
¼	to ½ pound of baby lettuce
1	bell pepper, chopped
½	cup chopped fresh parsley
½	cup chopped chives (optional)
	Salt and pepper to taste

DIRECTIONS

Marinate the mushrooms for 45 minutes in vinegar, olive oil, water, and sugar.

While mushrooms marinate, mix corn, tomatoes, onion, lettuce, pepper, parsley, chives, salt, and pepper in a large bowl.

Drizzle the marinated mushrooms over the salad or keep to the side and dip.

Grilled Vegetable Platter

Serves : 4

2 yellow bell peppers
2 red bell peppers
3 zucchini, halved lengthwise
3 squash, halved lengthwise
18 asparagus spears, tough ends trimmed
4 tomatoes

For dressing (*makes about 1 cup*) :
¾ cup olive oil
3 tbsp balsamic vinegar
2 cloves garlic, minced
1 tsp fresh lemon juice
Pinch dried basil
Pinch dried oregano
Salt and freshly ground pepper

DIRECTIONS

To make the dressing : Mix the ingredients together in a small bowl. Set aside.

Slice the vegetables and grill them over medium heat. Cook peppers until slightly charred. Cook zucchini and squash about 4 minutes on each side. Cook asparagus for about 5 minutes total. Cook tomatoes for about 3 minutes on each side.

Drizzle vegetables lightly with dressing.

Chilled Asparagus with Rosemary and Lemon Vinaigrette

Serves : 4-6

2 tsp fresh lemon juice
2 tbsp red wine vinegar
2 tbsp minced fresh rosemary
2 cloves garlic
1 tsp low-fat mayonnaise
½ cup extra virgin olive oil
Light sprinkle salt and pepper
30 asparagus spears, peeled
and tough ends trimmed

DIRECTIONS

Combine lemon juice, vinegar, rosemary, garlic, and mayonnaise in a small bowl. Whisk in the olive oil slowly to create a creamy sauce. Season with salt and pepper.

Bring a large sauté pan of water to a boil and add asparagus. Boil until tender. Remove the asparagus, then shock it in ice water (a gallon of water and three trays of ice) for about 2 minutes to stop the asparagus from cooking.

Drain asparagus again and place on paper towels and pat dry. Then arrange the asparagus on a serving platter. Cover and refrigerate about 1 hour until completely chilled.

When it's time to serve, pour vinaigrette evenly over the asparagus.

Tasty Tomatoes

Serves : 4-6

4	medium tomatoes
2	tsp minced chives
3	tbsp low-fat mayonnaise
1½	tsp Dijon mustard
	Light sprinkle salt and pepper
4	tbsp grated Parmesan cheese

DIRECTIONS

Preheat the oven to 375°F.

Cut tomatoes in half horizontally and place cut side up on a baking tray.

In a bowl, stir the topping : chives, mayonnaise, mustard, salt and pepper, and 2 tablespoons of the Parmesan cheese. Once the topping is nicely mixed, scoop out small amounts with a spoon and place on top of the tomatoes.

Take the rest of the cheese and sprinkle on top. Then bake for 10 minutes or until the tomatoes are hot. Once this is done, quickly put the tomatoes into the broiler for a minute to really get the topping brown and hot.

Serve hot.

WHAT WAS EASY IN PHASE I

WHAT WAS DIFFICULT IN PHASE I

PHASE II | Sample Recipes

NEW FOODS THAT YOU'VE COME TO LIKE

Breakfast | (*Phase II*)

Recipes on the go!

- 1 cup bran cereal
  1 cup low-fat milk
  1 medium banana
  1 cup orange juice

- 1½ cups puffed wheat
  1 cup low-fat milk
  ¼ cantaloupe

- 2 boiled eggs
  6-oz. cup plain yogurt
  1 cup low-fat milk

Lunch | (*Phase II*)

Kidney Beans with Sautéed Shrimp and Asparagus

Serves : 4

12 oz raw shrimp, peeled and deveined
1 tbsp olive oil
1 clove garlic, minced
3 cups kidney beans, cooked and drained, or use canned, rinsed beans
2 tbsp white wine
2 cups vegetable stock
2 cups steamed and chopped asparagus
1 tbsp minced fresh basil
1 tbsp minced fresh thyme
Salt and pepper to taste

For marinade :
2 tbsp fresh lemon juice
2 tsp minced fresh thyme
4 tbsp basil, cut into chiffonade (thin strips)
1 tbsp extra virgin olive oil
Salt and pepper to taste

DIRECTIONS

Combine marinade ingredients, add shrimp, and let stand in refrigerator for 20 minutes. Drain marinade and discard.

In a sauté pan, heat 1 tbsp olive oil over high heat and cook shrimp for 2 minutes per side.

Add garlic and briefly sweat until aromas are released.

Add kidney beans and white wine and cook for 1 minute over high heat.

Add the stock, bring to a simmer, and add the asparagus.

Heat through until all ingredients are hot and shrimp is a white, opaque color.

Remove from heat, add the fresh herbs, season to taste with salt and pepper, and serve.

NUTRITIONAL INFORMATION:

Per Serving : 429 Calories; 11g Fat (23.0% calories from fat); 33g Protein; 49g Carbohydrate; 12g Dietary Fiber; 131mg Cholesterol; 945mg Sodium. Exchanges: 3 Grain(Starch); 3 Lean Meat; 1/2 Vegetable; 0 Fruit; 2 Fat.

Greek Vegetable Stew with Garbanzo Beans

Serves : 4

1 tbsp olive oil
2 cups diced onion
1½ cups diced green bell pepper
2 cups sliced mushrooms
2 cups sliced artichoke hearts (can use frozen or canned if fresh is not available)
1 tsp cumin
1 pinch cinnamon
2 tbsp minced garlic
1½ quarts vegetable stock
3 cups Roma (plum) tomatoes, chopped
Salt and pepper to taste
2 cups garbanzo beans (chickpeas), cooked, or use canned, rinsed beans
1 tbsp lemon juice
⅓ cup Kalamata olives, pitted and sliced
1 tbsp minced fresh oregano
2 tbsp minced mint
2 tbsp minced dill
½ cup crumbled feta cheese

DIRECTIONS

In a sauté pan, heat olive oil over high heat and add onion, green pepper, mushrooms, artichokes, cumin, and cinnamon. Cook until golden brown, approximately 5 minutes, stirring occasionally.

Add garlic and stir. Cook for 20-30 seconds until the aromas are released.

Add stock and simmer for 15 minutes.

Add tomatoes and garbanzo beans and simmer for an additional 5 minutes.

Remove from heat. Add the lemon juice, olives, and herbs and serve in bowls, garnished with crumbled feta.

NUTRITIONAL INFORMATION:

Per Serving : 652 Calories; 22g Fat (28.7% calories from fat); 26g Protein; 96g Carbohydrate; 17g Dietary Fiber; 20mg Cholesterol; 3071mg Sodium. Exchanges: 4 Grain(Starch); 1 Lean Meat; 5 1/2 Vegetable; 0 Fruit; 4 Fat.

Seafood Gumbo with Brown Rice

Serves : 4

⅓ cup olive oil
⅓ cup whole wheat flour
1 cup diced onion
3 cloves garlic, minced
1 cup diced celery
1 cup diced green bell pepper
1 lb raw seafood, in any combination of fish or shrimp
3 tbsp filé powder
1 tsp cayenne pepper
1½ quarts vegetable stock
1½ cups okra
1 cup tomatoes
1 tbsp each fresh oregano, basil, and thyme
½ lb seafood or turkey sausage, cooked and sliced (optional)
Salt and pepper to taste
8 oz brown rice
1 quart water
Salt and pepper to taste

DIRECTIONS

In a large saucepan, heat olive oil over medium-low heat and add flour. Stir into a paste and cook for several minutes, stirring, until a rich nutty brown color develops. This mixture is called a "roux."

Add onion, garlic, celery, and green pepper to roux and cook for approximately 2 minutes, stirring constantly. Roux will cling to vegetables.

Add seafood and cook for approximately 3 minutes. Add filé powder and cayenne pepper. Add chicken stock and bring mixture to a simmer for ten minutes, stirring constantly.

Add okra, tomatoes, and herbs (and sausage if using) and cook for 5 minutes.

Season to taste with salt and pepper. Serve over brown rice.

To make brown rice, bring rice, 1 quart of water, and salt to a boil in an uncovered pot. Then reduce heat to low, cover, and simmer for approximately 45 minutes.

My Mother's Yummy Teriyaki Green Beans

Serves : 4

1 1-lb bag frozen green beans
2 tbsp olive oil
¼ cup of McCormick Grill Mates
teriyaki grilling sauce
1 cup Kikkoman stir-fry sauce
3 tbsp of House of Tsang
classic stir-fry sauce
2 shakes of Worcestershire sauce
2 shakes of soy sauce
2 shakes of Kikkoman
teriyaki sauce

DIRECTIONS

Heat oil until very hot.

Drop frozen beans into oil and turn immediately to coat beans with oil.

Add the remaining ingredients and stir until well coated.

Cook on low until tender, approximately 15 minutes.

Season to taste.

(Chopped Vegetable Salad)

Serves : 4-6

- 2 cucumbers, peeled and sliced
- 2 cups grape tomatoes, sliced in half
- 2 scallions, finely chopped (optional)
- 1 bell pepper, chopped
- 1 cup chopped fresh green beans
- ½ cup cooked corn
- 2 diced or thinly sliced carrots
- 2 tsp chives, minced

For dressing :

- ⅓ cup extra virgin olive oil
- ⅓ cup balsamic vinegar
- ½ tsp minced garlic
- Salt and pepper to taste

DIRECTIONS

Mix the cucumbers, tomatoes, scallions, pepper, beans, corn, carrots, and chives in a large bowl.

To make the dressing: In smaller bowl, mix oil, vinegar, garlic, salt, and pepper. Stir well.

Pour dressing over vegetables. Chill for fifteen minutes in refrigerator, then serve.

Dinner | (*Phase II*)

Garbanzo Beans with Chicken, Broccoli, and Tomato Broth

Serves : 4-6

2 tbsp fresh lemon juice
2 tsp minced fresh oregano
4 tbsp fresh basil, cut into chiffonade (thin strips)
1 tbsp extra virgin olive oil
Salt and pepper to taste
2 boneless, skinless chicken breasts, julienned
1 tbsp olive oil
1 clove garlic, minced
3 cups cooked garbanzo beans (chickpeas) or use canned, rinsed beans
2 cups broccoli, steamed and chopped

For tomato broth :

1 tbsp olive oil
¼ cup each diced carrot, onion, and celery
2 cloves garlic
1 tbsp white wine
3 Roma (plum) tomatoes, chopped
3 cups chicken broth
1 bay leaf
Basil stems (*from basil above*)
Salt and pepper to taste

DIRECTIONS

To make the tomato broth : Heat olive oil over medium heat and sweat carrots, onion, celery, and garlic cloves for approximately 2 minutes. Add white wine and cook for 1 minute. Add tomatoes, broth, bay leaf, and basil stems. Reduce heat and simmer for 20 minutes. Strain, season with salt and pepper, and set aside.

Combine lemon juice, 1 tsp of the oregano, 2 tsp of the basil, and the extra virgin olive oil. Add to chicken and let stand in refrigerator for 20 minutes. Drain.

To make the chicken : Heat 1 tbsp olive oil in a sauté pan over high heat and cook chicken until fully cooked (test one piece by cutting into it). Add garlic and briefly sweat until aromas are released.

Add garbanzo beans and cook for 1 minute over high heat. Add tomato broth, bring to a simmer, and add broccoli. Heat through until all ingredients are hot.

Remove from the heat, add remaining oregano and basil, season to taste with salt and pepper, and serve.

NUTRITIONAL INFORMATION:

Per Serving : 486 Calories; 15g Fat (28.9% calories from fat); 41g Protein; 45g Carbohydrate; 7g Dietary Fiber; 68mg Cholesterol; 1724mg Sodium. Exchanges: 2 Grain(starch); 4 1/2 Lean Meat; 1/2 Vegetables; 0 Fruit; 2 1/2 Fat.

Roasted Sea Bass

Serves : 4

- ½ cup fresh bread crumbs (optional for Phase II)
- 1 clove garlic, minced
- 3 tbsp chopped fresh parsley
- 2 tbsp minced fresh basil
- 2 tbsp drained capers (optional)
- 1 tsp Dijon mustard
- 1 tbsp fresh lemon juice
- Salt and freshly ground pepper to taste
- 3 tbsp extra virgin olive oil
- 4 4-oz. sea bass fillets without the skin

DIRECTIONS

Preheat the oven to 350°F.

Mix bread crumbs, garlic, parsley, basil, capers, mustard, lemon juice, salt, and pepper in a small bowl.

In a frying pan over high heat, sauté the sea bass in the oil for about 1-2 minutes on each side.

Apply the bread crumb mix to each fillet and make sure it adheres. Place the fillets on a rack set in a roasting pan.

Cook for about 10 minutes, to your preference.

WHAT WAS EASY IN PHASE II

WHAT WAS DIFFICULT IN PHASE II

PHASE III | Sample Recipes

ALL GOOD HABITS LEARNED IN PHASES I & 2

Recipes on the go!

- 1 English muffin, toasted
  2 tsp peanut butter
  6-oz cup plain low-fat yogurt
  ¾ cup blackberries

- ½ bagel, toasted
  4 egg whites
  1 cup fresh orange juice

- 2 eggs, scrambled
  1 English muffin
  1 tsp butter
  1 cup fresh orange juice

Country Breakfast Patty with Oatmeal and Side of Fruit

Serves : 4

8 oz ground turkey
2 eggs
2 tbsp diced red bell pepper
2 tbsp diced yellow onion
1 tsp minced fresh thyme
Salt and pepper to taste
1 tbsp olive oil
½ cup dry instant oats
1 cup skim milk
1 cup strawberries, sliced

DIRECTIONS

Combine ground turkey, eggs, pepper, onion, thyme, salt, and pepper and form into 4 patties.

Heat the olive oil in a sauté pan and sauté patties until cooked through and golden brown on both sides, approximately 3 minutes on each side, depending on the thickness of the patties.

Cook oats in milk according to package instructions.

Serve patty with side of sliced strawberries and oatmeal.

NUTRITIONAL INFORMATION:
Per Serving : 224 Calories; 11g Fat (46.1% calories from fat); 17g Protein; 13g Carbohydrate; 2g Dietary Fiber; 152mg Cholesterol; 223mg Sodium. Exchanges: 1/2 Grain(Starch); 2 Lean Meat; 0 Vegetable; 0 Fruit; 0 Nonfat Milk; 1 Fat.

Tropical Fruit Salad with Side of Turkey Sausage

Serves : 4

2 large turkey sausages
⅓ *cup each* :
Pineapple, peeled, cored, and chopped
Mango, pitted, peeled, and chopped
Papaya, pitted, peeled, and chopped
Banana, sliced
Strawberries, sliced
Kiwi, peeled and sliced
Mint leaves for garnish

DIRECTIONS

Preheat oven to 400°F.

To make the fruit salad : Combine fruit and toss.

Cook the turkey sausage in the oven for approximately 10 minutes or until done.

Cut sausages into halves and serve with fruit salad, garnished with mint leaf.

NUTRITIONAL INFORMATION:

Per Serving : 185 Calories; 11g Fat (52.8% calories from fat); 9g Protein; 14g Carbohydrate; 2g Dietary Fiber; 45mg Cholesterol; 382mg Sodium. Exchanges: 1 Lean Meat; 1 Fruit; 1 1/2 Fat.

Poached Eggs and Spinach on English Muffin with Tomato-Mint Coulis

Serves : 4

1 tsp olive oil
½ clove garlic, minced
1 tbsp diced onion
2 Roma (plum) tomatoes, roughly chopped
1 tsp red wine vinegar
Salt and pepper
1 tbsp minced mint
2 tsp distilled white vinegar
4 whole wheat English muffins, split
8 large eggs
2 cups spinach, steamed

DIRECTIONS

To make the coulis : In a saucepan, heat olive oil over medium heat and sweat garlic and onion until translucent. Add tomatoes and cook for 10 minutes. Add vinegar and simmer for an additional 2 minutes. Season to taste with salt and pepper, remove from heat, and puree in a food processor until smooth. Add fresh mint.

In a stockpot, bring one gallon of water and the white vinegar to a low simmer.

Toast the English muffins.

Carefully crack the eggs directly into the water and vinegar mixture, and let cook for 4 minutes. Remove them with a slotted spoon.

Spoon warm spinach over muffins, top with eggs, and spoon coulis over eggs.

NUTRITIONAL INFORMATION:

Per Serving : 311 Calories; 13g Fat (35.9% calories from fat); 19g Protein; 31g Carbohydrate; 5g Dietary Fiber; 424mg Cholesterol; 578mg Sodium. Exchanges: 1 1/2 Grain(Starch); 1 1/2 Lean Meat; 1/2 Vegetable; 1 Fat; 0 Other Carbohydrates.

Mushroom, Pepper, and Provolone Frittata with Macerated Fresh Berries

Serves : 4

For berries :

- 2 cups blueberries, strawberries, raspberries, and blackberries
- 1 tbsp granulated sugar substitute (Splenda recommended)
- 1 tbsp lemon juice

For frittata :

- 1 red bell pepper, diced
- 1 cup sliced mushrooms
- 1 tsp olive oil
- 4 large eggs
- 14 egg whites
- Salt and pepper to taste
- 4 thin slices provolone cheese
- 1 tbsp grated Parmesan cheese

DIRECTIONS

Preheat the oven to 500°F.

To macerate the berries : Toss them with the sugar substitute and lemon juice. Let stand while you make the frittata.

To make the frittata : In a small sauté pan, sauté red pepper and mushrooms in ½ teaspoon of the olive oil over high heat for about 2 minutes or until softened. Whisk together whole eggs and egg whites, and season to taste with salt and pepper.

In a separate oven-proof sauté pan, heat remaining olive oil over high heat and add eggs, stirring every minute for a total of approximately 5 minutes, or until eggs are set.

Layer the red pepper and mushrooms, provolone, and Parmesan on top of the omelet and place the pan in a 500°F oven or under the broiler for 2 minutes.

Cut into wedges and serve hot with the berries.

NUTRITIONAL INFORMATION:

Per Serving : 250 Calories; 11g Fat (38.6% calories from fat); 24g Protein; 14g Carbohydrate; 4g Dietary Fiber; 223mg Cholesterol; 418mg Sodium. Exchanges: 3 Lean Meat; 1/2 Vegetable; 1/2 Fruit; 1 Fat; 0 Other Carbohydrates.

Lunch | (*Phase III*)

Hearty Black Bean Soup

Serves : 8

- 1 lb black beans, soaked in water overnight or for at least 6 hours
- 2 medium onions, chopped
- 2 small carrots, chopped
- 1 celery stalk, chopped
- 4 tsp extra virgin olive oil
- 4 cloves garlic, minced
- ½ tsp dried oregano
- ½ tsp cumin
- 1 tsp soy sauce
- 1 tbsp fresh lemon juice

DIRECTIONS

Drain the beans. Put them on a large pot and add water to cover. Simmer beans until they are soft, about 1½ hours.

Sauté onion, celery, and carrot in olive oil. Add garlic, oregano, cumin, and soy sauce. Cook, stirring, for 5 minutes.

Add the vegetables to the beans.

Cook for another 30 minutes. Add more water if necessary.

Just before serving, add the lemon juice.

Chicken and Summer Vegetable Broth

Serves : 4

½ cup lentils
1 bay leaf, whole
2 quarts chicken stock
½ eggplant, diced
1 zucchini, diced
1 yellow squash, diced
1 red bell pepper, diced
½ cup Roma (plum) tomatoes, diced
½ cup green beans
Salt and pepper to taste
1 tbsp minced fresh basil
1 tsp minced fresh parsley
1 tsp minced fresh thyme

DIRECTIONS

Simmer lentils and bay leaf in chicken stock for 40 minutes.

Add the eggplant, zucchini, yellow squash, pepper, tomatoes, beans, salt, and pepper and simmer for 15 minutes.

Add fresh herbs and serve immediately.

NUTRITIONAL INFORMATION:

Per Serving : 171 Calories; 1g Fat (5.9% calories from fat); 11g Protein; 26g Carbohydrate; 11g Dietary Fiber; 0mg Cholesterol; 4304mg Sodium. Exchanges: 1 Grain(Starch); 1/2 Lean Meat; 2 Vegetable.

Dinner | (*Phase III*)

Black Beans with Herb-Marinated Chicken and Marinated Roasted Peppers

Serves : 4

2 boneless, skinless chicken breasts, julienned into strips
2 tbsp olive oil
1 tbsp minced fresh oregano
2 tbsp minced cilantro
3 tbsp lemon juice
1 tsp chili powder
1 tsp cumin
3 cups cooked black beans, or use canned, rinsed beans
2 red bell peppers, roasted, peeled, seeded, and sliced
1 green bell pepper, roasted, peeled, seeded, and sliced
1 yellow bell pepper, roasted, peeled, seeded, and sliced
⅓ cup pine nuts, toasted
2 cups chicken stock
Salt and pepper to taste

DIRECTIONS

To marinate the chicken breast : In a small bowl, combine half of the olive oil, oregano, cilantro, and lemon juice, and add all of the chili powder and cumin. Stir into the chicken.

Let the chicken stand in refrigerator for 20 minutes, then drain and discard marinade.

To cook the chicken, black beans, and pepper: Heat remaining olive oil in a sauté pan over high heat. Sauté chicken breast strips until cooked through.

Add beans and bell peppers, pine nuts, and chicken stock, and heat through until peppers are slightly cooked, about 2 minutes. Season with salt and pepper. Remove from heat, stir in remaining fresh herbs, and serve.

NUTRITIONAL INFORMATION:

Per Serving : 252 Calories; 7g Fat (24.6% calories from fat); 9g Protein; 40g Carbohydrate; 4g Dietary Fiber; 107mg Cholesterol; 614mg Sodium. Exchanges: 1 1/2 Grain(Starch); 1/2 Lean Meat; 1/2 Fruit; 0 Nonfat Milk; 1 Fat; 1/2 Other Carbohydrates.

Mahi-Mahi Satay with Lemongrass, Brown Rice, Snow Peas, and Ponzu Dipping Sauce

Serves : 4

For ponzu dipping sauce :

1 cup ponzu (Japanese citrus-base sauce available at supermarkets)
2 tbsp honey
1 tbsp chopped cilantro
1 tsp minced ginger
1 tsp minced scallion
1 tsp minced garlic
1 tsp sambal
(Asian hot sauce, available at supermarkets)
1 tbsp sesame oil

For rice :

⅔ cup short-grain brown rice
3 cups chicken stock
1 tbsp chopped scallion
1 tbsp minced lemongrass

For mahi-mahi satay :

4 4-oz portions mahi-mahi, cut into thin strips and skewered
2 cups snow peas
2 tbsp olive oil
1 tbsp soy sauce

DIRECTIONS

To make the ponzu dipping sauce : Combine ponzu, honey, cilantro, ginger, scallion, garlic, sambal, and sesame oil.

To make the rice : In a pot, combine rice, stock, scallion, and lemongrass. Bring to a boil, reduce heat, cover, and simmer for approximately 45 minutes or until the rice is cooked.

Heat an outdoor grill or a broiler.

To make the mahi-mahi satay : Marinate the mahi-mahi in one-quarter of the ponzu dipping sauce for 10 minutes. Place on the hot grill or in the broiler and cook for approximately 1½ minutes per side.

Heat olive oil in a wok or sauté pan over high heat. When oil begins to smoke, add snow peas and stir-fry for 2 minutes. Add soy sauce, mix in, and remove from heat. Serve the skewers over rice and snow peas with ponzu dipping sauce on the side.

NUTRITIONAL INFORMATION:

Per Serving : 374 Calories; 12g Fat (29.8% calories from fat); 25g Protein; 39g Carbohydrate; 2g Dietary Fiber; 49mg Cholesterol; 1934mg Sodium. Exchanges: 1 1/2 Grain(Starch); 2 1/2 Lean Meat; 1 Vegetable; 2 Fat; 1/2 Other Carbohydrates.

Chicken Marsala with Brown Rice Risotto and Sautéed Haricot Verts with Marinated Tomatoes

Serves : 4

For chicken :

¼ cup whole wheat flour
¼ cup olive oil
1 cup mushrooms, sliced
2 tbsp dry marsala
1½ cups chicken stock, warm
1 bay leaf
2 chicken breasts, sliced horizontally in 3 – 4 pieces
Salt and pepper to taste

For haricot verts :

2 tsp olive oil
2 cups haricot verts (thin French green beans)

DIRECTIONS

To make the chicken marsala : In a saucepan, heat 2 tablespoons olive oil and 2 tablespoons flour and cook, stirring, over medium heat until golden brown (this creates a nutty paste called a "roux"). Add mushrooms and cook for 3 minutes. Add marsala and cook for 1 minute. Add chicken stock and bay leaf, and simmer for 20 minutes. Dredge chicken breast strips in remaining whole wheat flour. Heat 2 tablespoons olive oil in a sauté pan over high heat and add chicken until cooked through. Drain oil from pan. Add marsala sauce and warm through, but do not continue to cook the chicken breast or it will become overcooked. Season with salt and pepper.

To make the haricot verts : Heat olive oil in a sauté pan over medium high heat. When oil is hot, add haricot verts and stir-fry for 3 minutes, remove from heat, and serve.

For risotto :

1 tsp olive oil
⅔ cup short-grain brown rice
¼ cup onion, diced
1 tbsp white wine
3 cups chicken stock
1 tsp extra virgin olive oil
1 tbsp grated Parmesan cheese (optional)

For marinated tomatoes :

4 Roma (plum) tomatoes, sliced ¼ inch thick
2 tbsp balsamic vinegar
1 tsp minced fresh oregano
1 tbsp fresh basil, cut into chiffonade (thin strips)
1 tsp extra virgin olive oil
Salt and pepper to taste

To make the risotto : Heat olive oil in saucepan over medium heat, then add onion and rice, and sweat for 2 minutes. Add white wine and cook for 1 minute, then add 1 cup chicken stock. Stir rice frequently. As liquid is absorbed and the bottom of the pan becomes visible, add another cup of stock, repeating until all the stock is absorbed and the rice is tender, approximately 45 minutes. Use water if all the stock is absorbed before the rice is cooked. Drizzle with extra virgin olive oil and add Parmesan if using.

To marinate the tomatoes : Combine all ingredients.

NUTRITIONAL INFORMATION:

Per Serving : 374 Calories; 12g Fat (29.8% calories from fat); 25g Protein; 39g Carbohydrate; 2g Dietary Fiber; 49mg Cholesterol; 1934mg Sodium. Exchanges: 1 1/2 Grain(Starch); 2 1/2 Lean Meat; 1 Vegetable; 2 Fat; 1/2 Other Carbohydrates.

Grilled Chicken Breast with Lentils, Creamless Cauliflower Gratin, and Jus

Serves : 4

For marinade :

2 tbsp fresh lemon juice
2 tsp chopped fresh oregano
4 tbsp fresh basil, cut into chiffonade (thin strips)
1 clove garlic
1 tbsp extra virgin olive oil
2 boneless, skinless chicken breasts, 7-8 oz each

For lentils :

1½ cups lentils (French lentils are recommended)
1 tbsp diced carrot
1 tbsp diced celery
1 tbsp diced onion
1 clove garlic, minced
1 tbsp diced mushrooms
1 tbsp olive oil
2 tbsp red wine
2½ cups chicken stock
1 bay leaf
Salt and pepper to taste

DIRECTIONS

Preheat the oven to 400°F. Prepare a grill or broiler for grilling the chicken.

To make the chicken : Combine marinade ingredients, add chicken, and let stand in refrigerator for 20 minutes. Drain and discard marinade. When lentils and cauliflower are almost ready, grill breasts over high heat or put under broiler until cooked through (approximtely 10 minutes). Slice the breasts and drizzle with the jus. Serve with the lentils and cauliflower.

To make the lentils : In a saucepan over medium heat, sweat lentils, carrot, celery, onion, garlic, and mushrooms in olive oil. Add red wine and cook for 2 minutes. Add chicken stock and bay leaf. Simmer until tender and liquid is absorbed, approximately 60-90 minutes. Remove bay leaf and serve.

For cauliflower gratin :

1 tbsp olive oil
½ onion, julienned
1 head cauliflower, sliced into ¼-inch-thick pieces
1 clove garlic, minced
1 tbsp white wine
1½ cups chicken stock
1 tbsp chopped parsley
2 tsp chopped fresh thyme
1 tbsp grated Parmesan cheese (optional)
Salt and pepper to taste

For jus :

1 tbsp diced carrot
1 tbsp diced celery
1 tbsp diced onion
½ tsp minced garlic
2 tsp olive oil
1 tbsp white wine
2½ cups chicken stock
1 bay leaf
Salt and pepper to taste

To make the cauliflower gratin : In an oven-proof sauté pan, heat olive oil over medium-low heat, add onion and cook until soft and caramelized, approximately 4 minutes. Add cauliflower and sweat for approximately 2 minutes. Add garlic and cook for approximately 30 seconds. Add wine and cook for approximately 1 minute. Add chicken stock, stir in parsley and thyme. Cover with foil and bake in 400°F oven for 20 minutes. Remove foil, sprinkle with Parmesan (if using) and place under broiler for approximately 5 minutes to brown on top.

To make the jus : Over medium heat, sweat the carrot, celery, onion, and garlic in olive oil. Add white wine and cook for 2 minutes. Add chicken stock and bay leaf. Simmer for 20 minutes and strain.

NUTRITIONAL INFORMATION:

Per Serving : 556 Calories; 15g Fat (25.5% calories from fat); 50g Protein; 49g Carbohydrate; 24g Dietary Fiber; 68mg Cholesterol; 3593mg Sodium. Exchanges: 3 Grain(Starch); 5 1/2 Lean Meat; 1 Vegetable; 0 Fruit; 2 1/2 Fat.

PHASE IV | Sample Recipes

Breakfast | (*Phase IV*)

Recipes on the go!

- 2 (4-inch) pancakes
  1 tbsp syrup
  ½ cup strawberries
  1 cup low-fat milk or
  orange or apple juice

- 1 mini bagel
  2 tsp jelly
  1 tbsp cream cheese
  1 cup low-fat milk or
  orange or apple juice

►►

- 2 slices whole wheat bread, toasted
  1 egg, scrambled
  1 tsp butter
  1 slice American cheese
  1 cup low-fat milk
  1 medium banana

- 2 low-fat waffles
  1 tsp syrup
  1 cup fresh orange juice
  1 cup low-fat yogurt

Blueberry Buckwheat Pancakes with Strawberry and Orange Compote

Serves : 4

For pancakes :

4 oz buckwheat flour
1 oz granulated sugar substitute (Splenda recommended)
2 tsp baking powder
½ tsp salt
2 large eggs, beaten
8 oz nonfat milk
½ cup blueberries
1 tbsp canola oil

For orange compote :

1 cup sliced strawberries
½ cup orange juice
1 tbsp granulated sugar substitute (Splenda recommended)

DIRECTIONS

To make the orange compote : Combine strawberries, orange juice, and sugar substitute and cook over low heat for 25 minutes. Let stand until warm or room temperature

To make the pancakes : Sift first four ingredients together into a medium mixing bowl. Add eggs, milk, and blueberries to dry ingredients. Do not overmix. Batter should remain slightly lumpy. Heat olive oil in nonstick pan or griddle over medium heat. Spoon 2-oz portions of pancake batter onto griddle. Cook for about 2 minutes or until edges become opaque and air bubbles on surface of pancakes begin to pop. Flip pancakes and cook for another 2 minutes.

Serve warm, drizzled with compote.

NUTRITIONAL INFORMATION:

Per Serving : 252 Calories; 7g Fat (24.6% calories from fat); 9g Protein; 40g Carbohydrate; 4g Dietary Fiber; 107mg Cholesterol; 614mg Sodium. Exchanges: 1 1/2 Grain(Starch); 1/2 Lean Meat; 1/2 Fruit; 0 Nonfat Milk; 1 Fat; 1/2 Other Carbohydrates.

Banana-Stuffed Whole Wheat French Toast with Mango Compote

Serves : 4

For French toast :

2 cups nonfat milk
1 large egg
1 tbsp granulated sugar substitute (Splenda recommended)
1 tsp cinnamon
2 tbsp canola oil
3 bananas, sliced thinly on the bias
8 slices whole wheat bread

For mango compote :

2 mangos, peeled, pitted, and diced
3 tbsp granulated sugar substitute (Splenda recommended)

DIRECTIONS

To make the mango compote : Combine mangos and sugar substitute and cook over low heat for 20 minutes. Let stand until warm or room temperature.

To make the French toast : Mix milk, egg, sugar substitute, and cinnamon. Heat olive oil in nonstick pan or griddle over medium heat. Distribute banana slices on four slices of bread, then gently press remaining four slices of bread on top of each bottom slice. Dip bread in milk and egg mixture, and cook over medium heat for about 3 minutes per side, or until golden.

Spoon mango compote over each serving.

NUTRITIONAL INFORMATION:

Per Serving : 399 Calories; 11g Fat (23.9% calories from fat); 12g Protein; 67g Carbohydrate; 7g Dietary Fiber; 55mg Cholesterol; 402mg Sodium. Exchanges: 1 1/2 Grain(Starch); 0 Lean Meat; 2 Fruit; 1/2 Nonfat Milk; 2 Fat; 1/2 Other Carbohydrates.

Egg White Omelet with Low-Fat Cheddar Cheese and Fresh Herbs

Serves : 4

18	egg whites
1	tsp minced fresh thyme
1	tsp minced fresh parsley
1	tsp minced fresh chives
	Salt and pepper to taste
2	tbsp olive oil
1½	cups shredded lowfat Cheddar cheese
½	cup sliced strawberries

DIRECTIONS

Whisk together egg whites, herbs, salt, and pepper.

In a nonstick omelet pan, heat one-quarter of the oil and pour in one-quarter of the egg white mixture.

Cook until set, stirring constantly with a rubber spatula.

Stir in one-quarter of the cheese, fold omelet over, and serve with side of strawberries.

Repeat for 3 more omelets.

NUTRITIONAL INFORMATION:

Per Serving : 215 Calories; 10g Fat (42.3% calories from fat); 26g Protein; 4g Carbohydrate; 1g Dietary Fiber; 9mg Cholesterol; 506mg Sodium. Exchanges: 0 Grain(Starch); 3 1/2 Lean Meat; 0 Vegetable; 0 Fruit; 1 1/2 Fat.

Dinner | (*Phase IV*)

Ahi Fish Tacos with Roasted Poblano Guacamole

Serves : 4

4 whole wheat tortillas

For tuna :

¼ tsp chili powder
¼ tsp cumin
¼ tsp dried oregano
Salt and pepper to taste
¼ tsp cayenne pepper
¼ tsp cinnamon
10 oz tuna steak, sliced 1/2-inch thick
1 tbsp olive oil
1 tbsp rice wine vinegar
1 tbsp lemon juice
2 tbsp hot sauce
1 cup shredded iceberg lettuce
1 red bell pepper, julienned
½ cup julienned red onion
¼ cup chopped fresh cilantro

DIRECTIONS

To make the tuna : Combine chili powder, cumin, dried oregano, salt and pepper, cayenne pepper, and cinnamon, and sprinkle on fish to season. In a sauté pan, heat oil over high heat. Sear tuna over very high heat (tuna should remain slightly pink in center). Combine vinegar, lemon juice, and hot sauce (any favorite variety) and toss with lettuce, bell pepper, red onion, and cilantro.

For guacamole :

1 small poblano pepper, roasted, peeled, and diced
1 small avocado, peeled and chopped
1 tsp lemon juice
1 clove garlic, minced
1 tbsp diced Roma (plum) tomato
1 tbsp diced red onion
1 tbsp minced cilantro
Salt and pepper to taste

To make the guacamole : Combine poblano pepper, avocado, lemon juice, garlic, tomato, red onion, cilantro, salt, and pepper and blend well.

To assemble : Place fish and vegetable mixture into tortillas, roll up, and cut tortillas in half.

Serve two halves per serving. Garnish with guacamole.

NUTRITIONAL INFORMATION:
Per Serving : 384 Calories; 17g Fat (39.5% calories from fat); 23g Protein; 37g Carbohydrate; 5g Dietary Fiber; 27mg Cholesterol; 695mg Sodium. Exchanges: 0 Grain(Starch); 2 1/2 Lean Meat; 1 Vegetable; 0 Fruit; 2 Fat; 0 Other Carbohydrates.

Roasted Chicken Breast with Brown Saffron Risotto, Oven-Dried Tomatoes, and Basil/Mint Jus

Serves : 4

For chicken breast :

2 boneless and skinless chicken breasts, 7-8 oz each
Salt and pepper to taste

For basil/mint jus :

1 tbsp diced carrot
1 tbsp diced celery
1 tbsp diced onion
½ tsp minced garlic
2 tsp olive oil
1 tbsp white wine
2½ cups chicken stock
2 sprigs fresh basil
2 sprigs fresh mint
1 bay leaf
Salt and pepper to taste

For oven-dried tomatoes :

16 Roma (plum) tomatoes, quartered (see shortcut substitution below)
1 tbsp olive oil

DIRECTIONS

Preheat oven to 400°F.

To roast the chicken breasts : Roast breasts in a 400°F oven until done, approximately 10 minutes. Let cool and slice into strips.

To make the basil/mint jus : Over medium heat, sweat carrot, celery, onion, and garlic in olive oil. Add white wine and cook for 2 minutes. Add chicken stock, basil, mint, and bay leaf. Simmer for 20 minutes. Season with salt and pepper. Strain.

To make the oven-dried tomatoes : Preheat oven to 225°F. Drizzle tomatoes with olive oil. Place in oven for 4 hours and remove. Let cool.
(Note substitution: You can use sun-dried tomatoes, simmered in water for 10 minutes and drained, then tossed with olive oil.)

For risotto :

2 tsp olive oil
2 tbsp yellow onion, peeled and diced
2 cups short-grain brown rice
1 tbsp white wine
7 cups chicken stock, hot
1 tbsp saffron
1 tsp extra virgin olive oil
Salt and pepper to taste
1 tbsp grated Parmesan cheese (optional)

To make the risotto : (Tip: Keep chicken stock simmering in a separate pot next to the risotto.) Heat olive oil in saucepan, over medium heat, add onion and rice, and sweat for 2 minutes. Add white wine and cook for 1 minute, then add 1 cup chicken stock and saffron. Stir rice frequently. As liquid is absorbed and the bottom of the pan is visible, add another cup of stock, repeating until all stock is absorbed, approximately 45 minutes. Drizzle with extra virgin olive oil and add Parmesan if using.

To serve : Spoon risotto into bowls and add tomatoes and chicken.

NUTRITIONAL INFORMATION:

Per Serving : 721 Calories; 15g Fat (19.6% calories from fat); 41g Protein; 99g Carbohydrate; 7g Dietary Fiber; 68mg Cholesterol; 5228mg Sodium. Exchanges: 5 Grain(Starch); 4 Lean Meat; 4 1/2 Vegetable; 2 Fat.

SNACKS:

ONLY CHOOSE ONE SNACK FOR THE ALLOTTED SNACK PERIOD IN YOUR EATING SCHEDULE. CHOOSE THE SNACK THAT FITS THE PHASE YOU'RE CURRENTLY IN.

- ⅓ cup plain low-fat yogurt dip and 2 cups raw vegetables
- Cashews (10)
- 2 graham cracker squares and 2 tsp low-sugar jelly
- 1 low-fat granola bar
- 15 grapes and ½ cup of low-fat milk
- ½ cup of plain low-fat yogurt
- 2 tbsp raisins and 10 peanuts
- 1 small brownie
- 2 gingersnaps and ½ oz cheddar cheese
- 1½ cups baby carrots
- 2 chocolate chip cookies, small (Oreo-sized)
- Tortilla chips, fat-free (15-20)
- ½ small pack of licorice
- Almonds (10-14)

- Jell-O Smoothie snacks (1 snack)
- 4 animal crackers and 1 small orange
- Popcorn, air-popped (3 cups, no butter!)
- 2 rice cakes topped with 1 tsp peanut butter
- 1 cup unsweetened applesauce
- Saltine crackers (7)
- 1 medium banana, frozen
- 8 halves dried apricots and ½ cup skim milk
- Sunflower seeds (2 tbsp)
- Sherbet (½ cup)
- ½ cup sugar-free chocolate pudding made with low-fat milk with 2 tbsp whipped topping
- Melba toast (4 slices)
- 6 saltine-type crackers topped with 2 tsp low-sugar jelly

DR. IAN'S TIP : Skip the power bars. They are convenient and attractively packaged, but are high in calories and sugar.

APPENDIX

Body Mass Index Chart

Fiber Content of Foods

How to Read a Food Label

Caloric Expenditure During Various Activities

BODY MASS INDEX (*BMI*)

Body Weight (pounds)

Height	18	19	20	21	22	23	24	25	26	27	28	29	30	31	32	33	34	35	36	37	38	39
4'10"	86	91	96	100	105	110	115	119	124	129	134	138	143	148	153	158	162	167	172	177	181	186
4'11"	89	94	99	104	109	114	119	124	128	133	138	143	148	153	158	163	168	173	178	183	188	193
5'0"	92	97	102	107	112	118	123	128	133	138	143	148	153	158	163	168	174	179	184	189	194	199
5'1"	95	100	106	111	116	122	127	132	137	143	148	153	158	164	169	174	180	185	190	195	201	206
5'2"	98	104	109	115	120	126	131	136	142	147	153	158	164	169	175	180	186	191	196	202	207	213
5'3"	102	107	113	118	124	130	135	141	146	152	158	163	169	175	180	186	191	197	203	208	214	220
5'4"	105	110	116	122	128	134	140	145	151	157	163	169	174	180	186	192	197	204	209	215	221	227
5'5"	108	114	120	126	132	138	144	150	156	162	168	174	180	186	192	198	204	210	216	222	228	234
5'6"	112	118	124	130	136	142	148	155	161	167	173	179	186	192	198	204	210	216	223	229	235	241
5'7"	115	121	127	134	140	146	153	159	166	172	178	185	191	198	204	211	217	223	230	236	242	249
5'8"	118	125	131	138	144	151	158	165	171	177	184	190	197	203	210	216	223	230	236	243	249	256
5'9"	122	128	135	142	149	155	162	169	176	182	189	196	203	209	216	223	230	236	243	250	257	263
5'10"	126	132	139	146	153	160	167	174	181	188	195	202	209	216	222	229	236	243	250	257	264	271
5'11"	129	136	143	150	157	165	172	179	186	193	200	208	215	222	229	236	243	250	257	265	272	279
6'0"	132	140	147	154	162	169	177	184	191	199	206	213	221	228	235	242	250	258	265	272	279	287
6'1"	136	144	151	159	166	174	182	189	197	204	212	219	227	235	242	250	257	265	272	280	288	295
6'2"	141	148	155	163	171	179	186	194	202	210	218	225	233	241	249	256	264	272	280	287	295	303
6'3"	144	152	160	168	176	184	192	200	208	216	224	232	240	248	256	264	272	279	287	295	303	311
6'4"	148	156	164	172	180	189	197	205	213	221	230	238	246	254	263	271	279	287	295	304	312	320
6'5"	151	160	168	176	185	193	202	210	218	227	235	244	252	261	269	277	286	294	303	311	319	328
6'6"	155	164	172	181	190	198	207	216	224	233	241	250	259	267	276	284	293	302	310	319	328	336

UNDERWEIGHT (<18.5) **HEALTHY WEIGHT** (18.5–24.9) **OVERWEIGHT** (25–29.9) **OBESE** (≥30)

Find your height along the left-hand column and look across the row until you find the number that is closest to your weight. The number at the top of that column identifies your BMI.

Source: From A. Must, G. E. Dallal, and W. H. Dietz, "Reference Data for Obesity: 85th and 95th Percentiles of Body Mass Index (wt/ht²) and Triceps Skinfold Thickness." *American Journal of Clinical Nutrition* 53 (1991): 839–846. Adapted with permission by the *American Journal of Clinical Nutrition*, © *American Journal of Clinical Nutrition*, American Society for Clinical Nutrition.

FIBER CONTENT OF FOODS

To consume more fiber, eat more whole fruits and vegetables, whole grains, and beans. Nuts are also rich in fiber, but they are energy dense, so eat them in small amounts. Use the following list to guide your food choices. It is adapted from research conducted by the Tufts University School of Medicine in Boston and published in the *Tufts Health & Nutrition Letter.*

FRUITS*	GRAMS OF FIBER
Apple (with skin)	4
Banana	3
Blueberries, ½ cup	2
Cantaloupe, 1 cup diced	1
Dates, ⅛ cup dry, chopped	2
Grapefruit, ½	2
Grapes, 1 cup	2
Nectarine (with skin)	2
Orange	3
Peach (with skin)	2
Pear (with skin)	4
Plum (with skin)	1
Prunes (dried), 10	2
Raisins, ⅛ cup	1
Raspberries, ½ cup	4
Strawberries, ½ cup	2
Watermelon, 1 cup diced	1

VEGETABLES†	GRAMS OF FIBER
Broccoli, ½ cup cooked, chopped	2
Broccoli, ½ cup chopped	1

*All values are for 1 medium-size fruit unless otherwise indicated.

†All values are for raw, uncooked vegetables unless otherwise indicated.

Brussels sprouts, ½ cup cooked	3
Carrot, 1 medium	2
Carrots, ½ cup cooked	3
Cauliflower, ½ cup cooked	2
Celery, 1 stalk	1
Corn, ½ cup cooked	2
Cucumber, ½ cup sliced	0.5
French fries, 1 small (2.5 ounces) serving	2
Green beans, ½ cup cooked (frozen)	2
Iceberg lettuce, 1 cup shredded	1
Peas, ½ cup cooked (frozen)	4
Peppers, ½ cup chopped	1
Potato, baked, with skin	5
Potato, baked, without skin	2
Potato, ½ cup mashed	2
Romaine lettuce, 1 cup shredded	1
Spinach, ½ cup chopped	1
Spinach, ½ cup cooked (frozen)	3
Sweet potato, baked with skin	3
Tomato, 1 medium	1

GRAINS, LEGUMES* (BEANS, CHICKPEAS, LENTILS, LIMA BEANS), AND NUTS	GRAMS OF FIBER
Black beans, ½ cup	8
Bread, 1 slice, white	1
Bread, 1 slice, whole-wheat	2
Bran muffin, 1 medium	3

*Values are for canned or cooked beans.

*(**Grains, Legumes, and Nuts**, continued)*	**GRAMS OF FIBER**
Chickpeas, ½ cup	5
Kidney beans, ½ cup	7
Lentils, ½ cup	8
Lima beans, ½ cup	6
Oatmeal, 1 cup cooked	4
Pasta, ½ cup cooked	1
Peanuts, ½ cup	6
Peanut butter, 2 tablespoons, chunky	2
Popcorn, 3 cups air-popped	2
Rice, 1 cup cooked, white	1
Rice, 1 cup cooked, brown	2
Sesame seeds, 2 tablespoons	1
Sunflower seeds, ⅛ cup	2
Tortilla chips, 1 cup (1.5 oz.)	1
Walnuts, ¼ cup chopped	2
Wheat germ, ¼ cup	4

HOW TO READ A FOOD LABEL

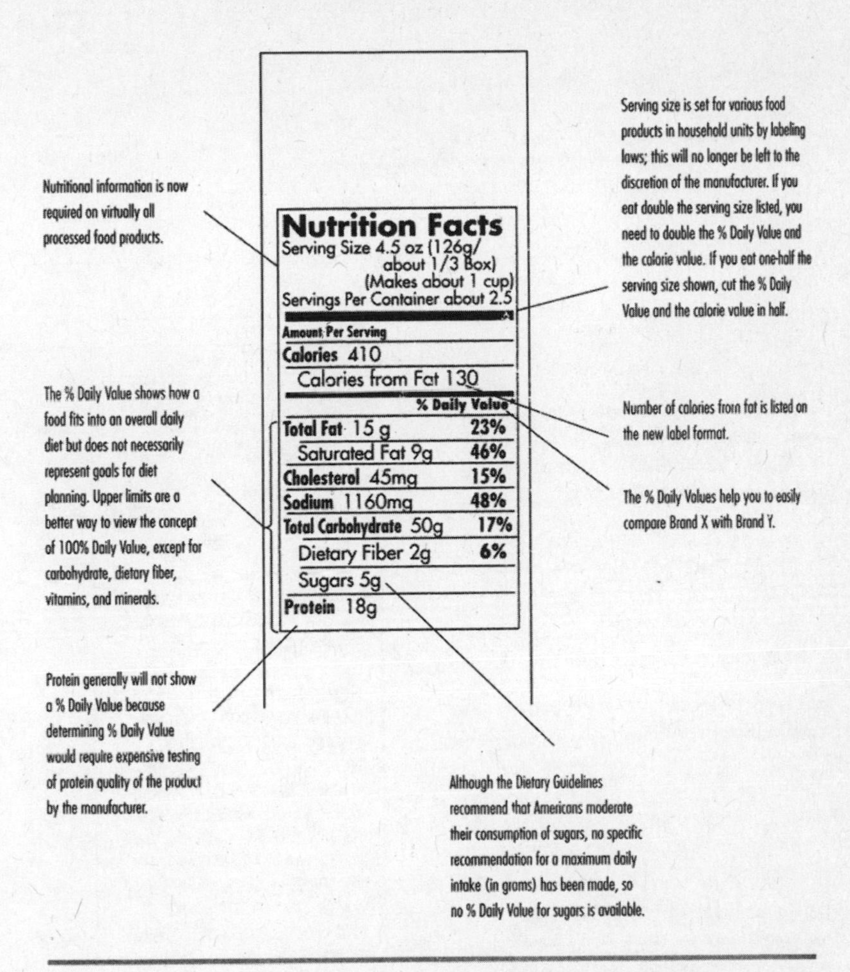

The Nutrition Facts panel on a current food label. The box is broken into two parts: A is the top, and B is the bottom. The % Daily Value listed on the label is the percentage of the generally accepted amount of a nutrient needed daily that is present in 1 serving of the product. You can use the % Daily Values to compare your diet with current nutrition recommendations for certain diet components. Let's consider dietary fiber. Assume that you consume 2,000 kcal. per day, which is the energy intake corresponding to the % Daily Values listed on labels. If the total % Daily Value for dietary fiber in all the foods you eat in one day adds up to 100%, your diet meets the recommendations for dietary fiber.

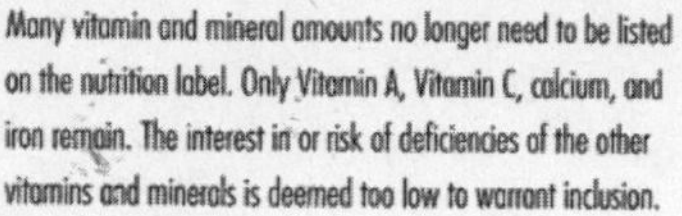

Many vitamin and mineral amounts no longer need to be listed on the nutrition label. Only Vitamin A, Vitamin C, calcium, and iron remain. The interest in or risk of deficiencies of the other vitamins and minerals is deemed too low to warrant inclusion.

Vitamin A 10% • Vitamin C 0%
Calcium 30% • Iron 15%

Some % Daily Value standards, such as grams of total fat, increase as energy intake increases. The % Daily Values on the label are based on a 2,000-kcal. diet. This is important to note if you don't consume at least 2,000 kcal. per day.

Percent Daily Values are based on a 2,000 calorie diet. Your daily values may be higher or lower depending on your calorie needs:

		Calories: 2,000	2,500
Total Fat	Less than	65g	80g
Sat Fat	Less than	20g	25g
Cholest	Less than	300mg	300mg
Sodium	Less than	2,400mg	2,400mg
Total Carb		300g	375g
Fiber		25g	30g

Labels on larger packages may list the number of calories per gram of fat, carbohydrate, and protein.

Calories per gram:
Fat 9 • Carbohydrate 4 • Protein 4

Ingredients, listed in descending order by weight, will appear here or in another place on the package. The sources of some ingredients, such as certain flavorings, will be stated by name to help people better identify ingredients that they avoid for health, religious, or other reasons.

INGREDIENTS: WATER, ENRICHED MACARONI (ENRICHED FLOUR [NIACIN, FERROUS SULFATE (IRON), THIAMINE MONONITRATE AND RIBOFLAVIN], EGG WHITE), FLOUR, CHEDDAR CHEESE (MILK, CHEESE CULTURE, SALT, ENZYME), SPICES, MARGARINE (PARTIALLY HYDROGENATED SOYBEAN OIL, WATER, SOY LECITHIN, MONO- AND DIGLYCERIDES, BETA CAROTENE FOR COLOR, VITAMIN A PALMITATE), AND MALTODEXTRIN.

Source: Wardlaw, Gordon M., *Contemporary Nutrition*, 4th ed. (New York: McGraw Hill Companies, Inc., 2000).

CALORIC EXPENDITURE DURING VARIOUS ACTIVITIES

ACTIVITY	CAL/MIN*
Sleeping	1.2
Resting in bed	1.3
Sitting, normally	1.3
Sitting, reading	1.3
Lying, quietly	1.3
Sitting, eating	1.5
Sitting, playing cards	1.5
Standing, normally	1.5
Classwork, lecture (listening)	1.7
Conversing	1.8
Personal toilet	2.0
Sitting, writing	2.6
Standing, light activity	2.6
Washing and dressing	2.6
Washing and shaving	2.6
Driving a car	2.8
Washing clothes	3.1
Walking indoors	3.1
Shining shoes	3.2
Making bed	3.4
Dressing	3.4
Showering	3.4
Driving motorcycle	3.4

*Depends on efficiency and body size. Add 10 percent for each 15 lb. over 150; subtract 10 percent for each 15 lb. under 150.

ACTIVITY	CAL/MIN
Metalworking	3.5
House painting	3.5
Cleaning windows	3.7
Carpentry	3.8
Farming chores	3.8
Sweeping floors	3.9
Plastering walls	4.1
Repairing trucks and automobiles	4.2
Ironing clothes	4.2
Farming, planting, hoeing, raking	4.7
Mixing cement	4.7
Mopping floors	4.9
Repaving roads	5.0
Gardening, weeding	5.6
Stacking lumber	5.8
Sawing with chain saw	6.2
Working with stone, masonry	6.3
Working with pick and shovel	6.7
Farming, haying, plowing with horse	6.7
Shoveling (miners)	6.8
Shoveling snow	7.5
Walking down stairs	7.1
Chopping wood	7.5
Sawing with crosscut saw	7.5–10.5
Tree felling (ax)	8.4–12.7
Gardening, digging	8.6
Walking up stairs	10.0–18.0
Playing pool or billiards	1.8
Canoeing, 2.5 mph–4.0 mph	3.0–7.0

ACTIVITY	CAL/MIN
Playing volleyball, recreational to competitive	3.5–8.0
Golfing, foursome to twosome	3.7–5.0
Pitching horseshoes	3.8
Playing baseball (except pitcher)	4.7
Playing Ping-Pong or table tennis	4.9–7.0
Practicing calisthenics	5.0
Rowing, pleasure to vigorous	5.0–15.0
Cycling, easy to hard	5.0–15.0
Skating, recreational to vigorous	5.0–15.0
Practicing archery	5.2
Playing badminton, recreational to competitive	5.2–10.0
Playing basketball, half or full court (more for fast break)	6.0–9.0
Bowling (while active)	7.0
Playing tennis, recreational to competitive	7.0–11.0
Waterskiing	8.0
Playing soccer	9.0
Snowshoeing (2.5 mph)	9.0
Slide board	9.0–13.0
Playing handball or squash	10.0
Mountain climbing	10.0–15.0
Skipping rope	10.0–15.0
Practicing judo or karate	13.0
Playing football (while active)	13.3
Wrestling	14.4
Skiing	
Moderate to steep	8.0–20.0

ACTIVITY	CAL/MIN
Downhill racing	16.5
Cross-country; 3–10 mph	9.0–20.0
Swimming	
Leisurely	6.0
Crawl, 25–50 yd/min.	6.0–12.5
Butterfly, 50 yd/min.	14.0
Backstroke, 25–50 yd/min.	6.0–12.5
Breaststroke, 25–50 yd/min.	6.0–12.5
Sidestroke, 40 yd/min.	11.0
Dancing	
Modern, moderate to vigorous	4.2–5.7
Ballroom, waltz to rumba	5.7–7.0
Square	7.7
Walking	
Road or field (3.5 mph)	5.6–7.0
Snow, hard to soft (2.5–3.5 mph)	10.0–20.0
Uphill, 15 percent grade (3.5 mph)	8.0–15.0
Downhill, 5–10 percent grade (2.5 mph)	3.5–3.7
15–20 percent grade (2.5 mph)	3.7–4.3
Hiking, 40-lb. pack (3.0 mph)	6.8
Running	
12-min. mile (5 mph)	10.0
8-min. mile (7.5 mph)	15.0
6-min. mile (10 mph)	20.0
5-min. mile (12 mph)	25.0

Source: Sharkey, Brian J., PhD., *Fitness and Health*, 4th ed. (Champaign: Human Kinetics, 1997).

BIBLIOGRAPHY

Books

Atkins, Robert C., M.D., *Dr. Atkin's Diet Revolution* (New York: Bantam, 1972).

Brody, Tom, *Nutritional Biochemistry,* 2nd ed (Academic Press, 1999).

Cooper, Kenneth H., M.D., M.PH., *The Aerobics Program for Total Well-Being* (New York: Bantam Books, 1982).

Hensrud, Donald D., M.D., *Mayo Clinic on Healthy Weight* (New York: Kensington Publishing Corporation, 2000).

Katch, Frank I., and McArdle, William D., *Introduction to Nutrition, Exercise, and Health,* 4th ed. (Baltimore: Lippincott Williams and Wilkins, 1988).

Mathews, Christopher K., and van Holde, K. E., *Biochemistry* (Redwood City, Calif.: Benjamin/Cummings Publishing Company, 1990).

McArdle, William D., Katch, Frank I., and Katch, Victor L., *Exercise Physiology: Energy, Nutrition, and Human Performance,* 4th ed. (New York: Lippincott Williams and Wilkins, 1996).

Paulsen, Barbara, *The Diet Advisor* (New York: Time-Life Books, 2000).

Rolls, Barbara, Ph.D., and Barnett, Robert, *Volumetrics Weight-Control Plan* (New York: HarperCollins, 2000).

Sears, Barry, Ph.D., *The Zone* (New York: HarperCollins, 1995).

Sharkey, Brian J., PhD., *Fitness and Health,* 4th ed. (Champaign: Human Kinetics, 1997).

Sizer, Frances, and Whitney, Eleanor, *Nutrition: Concepts and Controversies,* 8th ed. (Stamford: Wadsworth/Thomson Learning, 2000).

Steward, H. Leighton, Bethea, Morrison C., Nadrews, Sam S., Brennan, Ralph O., and Balart, Luis A. , *Sugar Busters!: Cut Sugar to Trim Fat* (New York: Ballantine, 1998).

Tarnower, Herman, and Baker, Samm Sinclair *Complete Scarsdale Medical Diet*

Plus Dr. Tarnower's Lifetime Keep-Slim Program (New York: Bantam Books, 1995).

Wardlaw, Gordon M., *Contemporary Nutrition: Issues and Insights*, 4th ed. (New York: The McGraw-Hill Companies, Inc., 2000).

Studies/Articles

The American Dietetics' Association Food and Nutrition Guide.

Willett, W.C., Dietz, W. H., and Colditz, G. A., "Guidelines for Healthy Weight," *New England Journal of Medicine* 341 (1999): 427–34.

National Institutes of Health, "Clinical Guidelines on the Identification, Evaluation, and Treatment of Overweight and Obesity in Adults" (September 1998).

U.S. Department of Health and Human Services, "Physical Activity and Health: A Report of the Surgeon General" (Atlanta, GA.: Centers for Disease Control and Prevention, National Center for Chronic Disease Prevention and Health Promotion, 1996).

Paffenbarger, R. S., Hyde, R. T., Wing, A. L., et al., "The Association of Changes in Physical-Activity Level and Other Lifestyle Characteristics with Mortality Among Men," *New England Journal of Medicine* 328, no. 8 (1993): 538–45.

Sherman, S. E., D'Agostino, R. B., Cobb, J. L., et al., "Physical Activity and Mortality in Women in the Framingham Heart Study," *American Heart Journal* 128, no. 5 (1994): 879–84.

Pate, R. R., Pratt, M., Blair, S. N., et al. "Physical Activity and Public Health: A Recommendation from the Centers for Disease Control and Prevention and the American College of Sports Medicine," *Journal of the American Medical Association* 273, no. 5 (1995): 402–407.

USDA and U.S. Department of Health and Human Services, *Dietary Guidelines for Americans*, 5th ed. (USDA Home and Garden Bulletin No. 232. Washington, D.C.: USDA, 2000).

USDA, *The Food Guide Pyramid* (USDA Home and Garden Bulletin No. 252. Washington, D.C.: USDA, 1992).

Flegal, K. M., Carroll, M.D., Kuczmarski, R. J., et al, "Overweight and Obesity in the United States: Prevalence and Trends, 1960–1994," *International Journal of Obesity* 22, no. 1 (1998): 39–47.

NIH, "Clinical Guideline on the Identification, Evaluation and Treatment of Overweight and Obesity in Adults—The Evidence Report," *Obesity Research* 6 (suppl. 2, 1998): 51S–209S.

PHS, *The Surgeon General's Report on Nutrition and Health* (DHHS Pub. No. [PHS] 88050210, Washington, D.C.: HHS, 1988).

INDEX

ABOUT THE AUTHOR

Dr. Ian Smith is a medical contributor to ABC's nationally syndicated *The View*, a medical columnist for *Men's Health* magazine, and the medical/diet expert on VH1's *Celebrity Fit Club*. Dr. Smith is also the host of the nationally syndicated radio show *Healthwise* on American Urban Radio Networks. He was formerly a medical correspondent for NBC News and for NewsChannel 4, where he filed reports for NBC's *Nightly News* and the *Today* show as well as WNBC's news broadcasts. He has written for a variety of publications including *Time*, *Newsweek*, and the New York *Daily News*, and has been featured in *People*, *Essence*, *Ebony*, *Cosmopolitan*, and *University of Chicago Medicine on the Midway*.

Dr. Smith graduated from Harvard College with an AB and received a master's in science education from Columbia University. He attended Dartmouth Medical School and completed the last two years of his medical education at the University of Chicago Pritzker School of Medicine.

Dr. Smith is also the author of three other books: *The Blackbird Papers: A Novel* (2005 BCALA fiction Honor Book Award winner), *Dr. Ian Smith's Guide to Medical Websites,* and *The Take-Control Diet.*